Female genital mutilation

• • • • • • • • • • • • • •

An overview

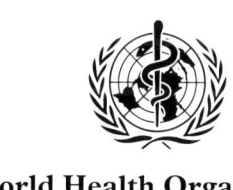

World Health Organization
Geneva
1998

WHO Library Cataloguing in Publication Data

Female genital mutilation : an overview.
   1. Circumcision, Female 2. Public policy 3. Human rights
   ISBN 92 4 156191 2   (NLM Classification: WP 200)

The World Health Organization welcomes requests for permission to reproduce or translate its publications, in part or in full. Applications and enquiries should be addressed to the Office of Publications, World Health Organization, Geneva, Switzerland, which will be glad to provide the latest information on any changes made to the text, plans for new editions, and reprints and translations already available.

© World Health Organization, 1998

Publications of the World Health Organization enjoy copyright protection in accordance with the provisions of Protocol 2 of the Universal Copyright Convention. All rights reserved.

The designations employed and the presentation of the material in this publication do not imply the expression of any opinion whatsoever on the part of the Secretariat of the World Health Organization concerning the legal status of any country, territory, city or area or of its authorities, or concerning the delimitation of its frontiers or boundaries.

The mention of specific companies or of certain manufacturers' products does not imply that they are endorsed or recommended by the World Health Organization in preference to others of a similar nature that are not mentioned. Errors and omissions excepted, the names of proprietary products are distinguished by initial capital letters.

The authors alone are responsible for the views expressed in this publication.

Designed by WHO Graphics
Typeset and printed in Switzerland
98 / 11931 - Strategic / Schuler - 9500

Contents

Foreword	v
Acknowledgements	vi
Introduction	vii

1. Definitions and classifications 1
    Background 1
    Early classifications 3
    Current WHO classification 5
    Description of the different types of female genital mutilation 6

2. Prevalence and epidemiology 9
    Background 9
    Africa 10
    Refugee and immigrant populations 18
    Evidence of prevalence in other regions 21

3. Health consequences 23
    Development and functional anatomy of the external
        female genitalia 23
    Physical consequences and complications 25
    Psychological and sexual effects 31

4. Research 37
    Past research 37
    Suggested research agenda 38

**5. International, regional and national
    agreements and actions** 50
    International 50
    Regional 55

National	56
Ethical considerations	57
6. WHO policies and activities	**59**
7. Conclusion	**63**
References	66
Recommended further reading	73

Foreword

Female genital mutilation, a traditional practice that can have serious health consequences, is of great concern to the World Health Organization (WHO). In addition to causing pain and suffering, it is a violation of internationally accepted human rights.

In the last few years, WHO's governing bodies have adopted a number of resolutions urging Member States to establish clear national policies to end traditional practices that are harmful to the health of women and children and requesting WHO to strengthen its technical support and other assistance to the countries directly concerned. Activities are being carried out to combat this practice as part of WHO's broader programmes on women's and children's health.

WHO has consistently and unequivocally advised that female genital mutilation, in any of its forms, should not be practised by any health professionals in any setting — including hospitals or other health establishments. While recognizing that female genital mutilation is an important reproductive health issue, it is also a sensitive topic. The issue must be approached with an understanding of the context of the cultural practice and its meaning for communities that practise it.

Much has already been achieved in the last decade in lifting the veil of secrecy from female genital mutilation and developing a strategy to bring about changes. However, there are still major gaps in understanding the extent of the problem, its health impact and the kinds of interventions that can be successful in eliminating it.

Lack of information hampers work in this area. This is why WHO is focusing on increasing knowledge and promoting technically sound policies and approaches to eliminate female genital mutilation.

This review, which includes an assessment of the epidemiological status and health complications of female genital mutilation and past and present policies at international, regional and national levels, aims to assist government agencies and nongovernmental organizations that are working to eliminate this practice. We hope that the book will help to turn this challenge into an opportunity for change in the lives of women.

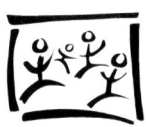
Dr Tomris Türmen
Executive Director
Family and Reproductive Health
World Health Organization

Acknowledgements

This publication has been prepared by N. Toubia and S. Izett of RAINB♀ Research, Action and Information Network for Bodily Integrity of Women.

The authors wish to acknowledge the contribution of Ms Elizabeth Kiberger who researched and helped draft legal and policy information. The contribution of the staff of the World Health Organization Family and Reproductive Health programme is also gratefully acknowledged.

Introduction

The traditional practice of female genital mutilation, sometimes referred to as female circumcision, has attracted increasing international attention in the past 20 years. Activists and nongovernmental organizations (NGOs) have used the opportunity provided by world conferences organized by the United Nations,[1] together with associated nongovernmental forums, to establish a strong global consensus against this practice and to consolidate the will and resources of national, regional and international institutions to stop it. WHO has been the leading United Nations specialized agency to take a position against female genital mutilation, starting in the 1960s. It is coordinating action in this area with the United Nations Children's Fund (UNICEF) and the United Nations Population Fund (UNFPA). In April 1997, WHO, UNICEF and UNFPA issued a joint statement expressing their common purpose in supporting the efforts of governments and communities to promote and strengthen action for the elimination of female genital mutilation. In recent years, increasing recognition of the human rights of women and children has brought additional calls for the practice to be stopped.

This book is intended primarily to document the medical and health facts about female genital mutilation together with related information as it appeared in the published literature, both formally in peer-reviewed journals and informally in country reports and publications resulting from workshops and conferences over the years. The book also considers legislation, human rights declarations and other action relevant to efforts to combat this practice. A special effort has been made to review past research in order to identify gaps in knowledge and make recommendations for future research priorities.

---

[1] World Conferences on Women, Copenhagen, 1980, Nairobi, 1985, Beijing, 1995; World Conference on Human Rights, Vienna, 1993; International Conference on Population and Development, Cairo, 1994; World Summit for Social Development, Copenhagen, 1995.

This is not a comprehensive review of all aspects of female genital mutilation. Many organizations and countries have developed projects to educate communities or to change attitudes and behaviours towards this practice. These projects are not adequately documented and any attempt to list them would be an arduous task. Evaluation of the success or failure of these efforts is also extremely difficult at this stage. However, the walls of silence surrounding the practice have been broken. There is more willingness by all concerned to face the problem. This is the first step towards creating conditions conducive to behavioural change with regard to female genital mutilation and is a major breakthrough. Although more work needs to be done, this achievement should be acknowledged. Some communities known to practise female genital mutilation have migrated to other countries. However, little is known about the numbers of girls who have undergone female genital mutilation or who are at risk of female genital mutilation in the new communities. Although several countries have passed laws against the practice, many now recognize that laws alone are not effective and are increasingly supporting preventive education programmes within the communities directly concerned. The increasing involvement of WHO and other technical agencies in this complex area of women's health will not only add to the visibility of the issue but will strengthen work that has already begun.

This book is intended primarily to address many of the scientific and medical questions related to female genital mutilation. It is hoped that it will prove useful not only to health professionals as they consider their role in relation to this practice but also to other individuals and groups active in combating female genital mutilation or in a position to develop policies and take action to stop it. Readers may not find all the answers to their questions or concerns here. However, the list of references gives direction for further investigations.

The review has been prepared by Nahid Toubia and Susan Izett of RAINB♀ — Research and Information Network for Bodily Integrity of Women. This nongovernmental body is well known for its commitment to the protection and promotion of the health of women and girls, and in particular to the elimination of female genital mutilation.

1.
Definitions and classifications

Background

Both traditional and modern genital surgery is performed in different societies for a variety of medical, cosmetic, psychological or social reasons. The surgical procedures included in the definition of female genital mutilation used in this book are limited to cutting rituals performed exclusively for cultural and traditional reasons on girls or young women, often without their approval or full understanding of the consequences of the procedures.[1] The procedures are outlined in the current WHO definition and classification of female genital mutilation which is reproduced on page 6. Surgeries described in the medical literature as circumcision for treatment of sexual disorders[2] and sex-determining surgeries for hermaphroditism[3] are

---

[1] The issue of consent by an individual of majority age (adult) to non-therapeutic surgery or any physical or psychological act by another, which may be perceived by some as a violation, is a widely debated and controversial issue which is not considered in depth in this review. The authority and limitation of parents and guardians to consent or withhold consent on behalf of a minor for treatment or surgery, whether medical or ritualistic, is a subject that requires more comprehensive discussion in the future. For further reading on these issues see, for example, Katz, 1984 *(1)* and Anderson, 1993 *(2)*. Also refer to principles established in the World Medical Association Declarations of Geneva (1948), Helsinki (1964) and Tokyo (1975) *(3-5)*.

[2] Medically prescribed "circumcisions" allegedly treat women for decreased sexual response or "frigidity". These operations usually involve the removal of the prepuce or foreskin from around the glans clitoris of adult women to increase exposure of the sensitive area. This procedure may be categorized as plastic surgery and is therefore beyond the scope of discussion of this review. Other genital cosmetic surgeries, involving trimming of the labia or repositioning of the clitoris, are reported in parts of Europe and North America *(6, p.107)*. Such operations were performed in Norway in the recent past on women with wide inner lips colloquially termed "bat lips". The law against female genital mutilation which was passed in Norway in 1995 also outlawed this operation. Apart from this one exception, such operations are legal in most countries on the basis that, like all cosmetic surgeries, they are requested by adult women legally capable of consent. The question of the nature of consent when culture is a major determining factor in women's choices is an important one but is also beyond the scope of this work.

[3] In sex-determining surgeries for hermaphroditism, one set of gonads is removed and there is some form of plastic reconstruction of the external genitals, which may involve amputation of some parts. One of the objections to such procedures is that they are performed on non-consenting children.

excluded. However, the limitations set for the purposes of this book should not preclude future discussions and appropriate scientific debate to expand or limit criteria for what constitutes female genital mutilation.

Female genital mutilation is mostly performed as a rite of passage from childhood to adulthood and is undertaken in most communities between the ages of four and 14 years. However, the age varies from area to area. For example, in southern Nigeria female genital mutilation is performed on babies in the first few months of life while in Uganda it is performed on young adult women. It is difficult to summarize the cultural significance of the practice in a few sentences because the cultures in which it occurs are very diverse. The reasons and meaning mostly revolve around social definitions of femininity and attitudes towards women's sexuality. A common feature is the social conditioning of women to accept female genital mutilation within social definitions of womanhood and identity. This leads them to perpetuate and defend the practice. Although many of these societies acknowledge the dampening effect of genital mutilation on women's sexual pleasure, preservation of chastity is not always the goal. In Egypt, Somalia and Sudan, for example, extramarital sex is completely unacceptable and female genital mutilation is used to ensure that it does not occur. In Kenya, Uganda and west African countries such as Sierra Leone, a girl may have a child out of wedlock to prove her fertility, then undergo genital mutilation and be married afterwards. For a mother in a society where there is little economic viability for women outside marriage, ensuring that a daughter undergoes genital mutilation as a child or teenager is a loving act to make certain of her marriageability. Because of the very private nature of the practice, the operation is performed at the request of the family and condoned by society as part of its cultural identity. The roots of the practice run deep into the individual's psychology, sense of loyalty to family and belief in a value system. These aspects are discussed further in section 3.

Controversy continues over the use of the terms "female circumcision" and "female genital mutilation" to describe the procedures employed. "Female circumcision" appeared in the reports of explorers and missionaries in Africa as early as the late nineteenth century and continued to be used until the 1980s. The term "female genital mutilation", used in the 1980s mostly by western writers (7), was endorsed by the Inter-African Committee on Traditional Practices Affecting the Health of Women and Children (IAC) during its regional meeting in 1989 (unpublished report).

The most common argument over the term "female circumcision" relates to whether or not the procedure is analogous to male circumcision. In the medical literature, "circumcision" is used specifically to mean removing the prepuce or foreskin of the penis or the clitoris. In young girls

1. DEFINITIONS AND CLASSIFICATIONS

this procedure is extremely difficult to perform. However, in general use the term is not so precise and merely describes ritualistic cutting of the genitals for cultural or religious reasons. In the latter sense, "female circumcision" is no different from male circumcision, as both are cutting rituals performed on a child with no demonstrated positive impact on health. One difference between the two practices is that male circumcision is a clear requirement of some religions while "female circumcision" is not. The most important difference, however, is that even the most minimal form of "female circumcision" can affect a girl's normal sexual function. Evidence in the medical literature on the effect of circumcision on male sexual function is not as yet well established.[1]

The most common types of female genital cutting rituals involve amputation of part or all of the clitoris and the labia minora resulting in irreparable physical damage and increased risk of health complications (the anatomy of the external female genitalia and the effects of female genital mutilation on health are described in section 3). It is because of the severity and irreversibility of the damage inflicted on the girl's body that the procedure has been termed "female genital mutilation", often abbreviated to FGM. This is currently the term used in all official documents of the United Nations and in the documents of world conferences such as the Programme of Action of the International Conference on Population and Development, 1994 (*9*), and the Declaration and Platform for Action of the Fourth World Conference on Women, 1995 (*10*). Its use has also been endorsed by WHO (*11*). In this book "female genital mutilation" is used except when quoting a source in which the term "female circumcision" is used.

Early classifications

A review of the literature reveals a wide range of terminology and descriptions of types and classifications of female genital mutilation. The first recorded attempt at classification was put forward by Daniell in 1847 (*12*). He described four types of clitoridectomy and excisions of labia in West Africa but did not mention any stitching of the vulva. Roles (*13*) in his review of anthropological literature of the nineteenth century described the ritual in East Africa as comprising three types: clitoridectomy, clitoridectomy and removal of the labia minora, and clitoridectomy with removal of the labia minora and majora.

---

[1] For further discussion of this subject, please see, for example, Taylor, Lockwood & Taylor, 1996 (*8*).

Worsley (*14*), who worked in a maternity hospital in Sudan in the 1930s, also wrote of three types:

> "a) introcision, or cutting into the vagina at an early age; b) the circumcision of women, paring the edges of the labia, together with excision of the clitoris; and c) infibulation proper, which is the aforementioned circumcision, but followed by almost complete closure of the vulval orifice".

Introcision was described by the British, when they entered Australia, as being a part of the complex initiation rituals of both sexes among some Aboriginal tribes. These rituals varied by region and introcision was not uniformly present among all subgroups. Worsley reported (*14*) that it was practised among the Petta-Petta tribe in the following manner:

> "When the girl reaches puberty, the whole tribe, of both sexes, is assembled. The operator, an elderly man trained for the purpose, enlarges the vaginal orifice by tearing it downwards with three fingers bound round with opossum string. In other districts the perineum is split up with a stone knife. This is usually followed by compulsory intercourse with a number of young men, and... [other practices] for the rejuvenation of the tribal aged and infirm."

In contemporary literature, Shandall (*15*) put forward a much-quoted classification in 1967, based on one of the earliest clinical studies of a large sample of "circumcised" women, which describes four types:

> "Type 1: Circumcision proper. This is the circumferential excision of the clitoral prepuce and is clearly analogous to male circumcision. In Muslim countries it is known as Sunna circumcision.
>
> Type 2: Excision. Besides the prepuce, this involves the removal of the glans clitoridis or even the clitoris itself and may include part, or the whole, of the labia minora.
>
> Type 3: Infibulation. This is also called Pharaonic circumcision. It involves partial closure of the vaginal orifice after excision of a varying amount of vulval tissue. In its drastic form, all or part of the mons veneris, labia majora and minora, and the clitoris are removed and the raw areas left to heal across the lower end of the vagina. After the operation, the thighs are strapped together and kept so for 40 days, complete occlusion of the introitus being prevented by the insertion of a small sliver of wood commonly a match-stick.
>
> Type 4: Introcision. This is the cutting into the vagina or splitting of the perineum, either digitally or by means of a sharp instrument, and is the severest form of circumcision."

1. DEFINITIONS AND CLASSIFICATIONS

These types correspond to those put forward by Verzin (*16*) in 1975. This classification was more accurate than the previous ones but still had several drawbacks, namely:

- The existence of a ritual operation which can be classified as type 1 or "true circumcision" has never been adequately documented. What is locally referred to as Sunna circumcision in many countries often includes removal of part or all of the clitoris, as is the case in Egypt and Sudan.

- The term "Pharaonic" is a Sudanese colloquial reference to infibulation and also implies a historical origin which is still open to question. The same type of female genital mutilation is referred to as "Sudanese circumcision" in Egypt. The use of colloquial terminology in the literature without reference to a standardized scientifically-based classification has resulted in confusion when comparing reports from different countries.

- Including introcision in a formal classification is not useful. There is no evidence of this practice outside Australia, either in Sudan or other African countries that practice female genital mutilation. A recent inquiry to the Australian government revealed that there are no known reports of the practice currently among the indigenous population (unpublished communication).

Many modifications of the Shandall classifications followed, adding further to the confusion (*16–22*).

Current WHO classification

Recognizing the need for a standardized classification, WHO convened a Technical Working Group on Female Genital Mutilation in Geneva, Switzerland, in July 1995. That Technical Working Group described the practice, and WHO's attitude to it, as follows (*11*):

> "Female genital mutilation is a deeply rooted, traditional practice. However, it is a form of violence against girls and women that has serious physical and psychosocial consequences which adversely affect health. Furthermore, it is a reflection of discrimination against women and girls.

> WHO is committed to the abolition of all forms of female genital mutilation. It affirms the need for the effective protection and promotion of the human rights of girls and women, including their rights to bodily integrity and to the highest attainable standard of physical, mental and social well-being.

WHO strongly condemns the medicalization of female genital mutilation, that is, the involvement of health professionals in any form of female genital mutilation in any setting, including hospitals or other health establishments."

The joint statement on female genital mutilation issued in April 1997 by WHO, UNICEF and UNFPA gave the following definition to the practice (23):

"Female genital mutilation comprises all procedures involving partial or total removal of the external female genitalia or other injury to the female genital organs whethe<<r for cultural or other non-therapeutic reasons."

The three agencies classified the different types of female genital mutilation as follows:

Type I   Excision of the prepuce, with or without excision of part or all of the clitoris.

Type II   Excision of the clitoris with partial or total excision of the labia minora.

Type III   Excision of part or all of the external genitalia and stitching/narrowing of the vaginal opening (infibulation).

Type IV   Unclassified: includes pricking, piercing or incising of the clitoris and/or labia; stretching of the clitoris and/or labia; cauterization by burning of the clitoris and surrounding tissue; scraping of tissue surrounding the vaginal orifice (angurya cuts) or cutting of the vagina (gishiri cuts); introduction of corrosive substances or herbs into the vagina to cause bleeding or for the purposes of tightening or narrowing it; and any other procedure that falls under the definition of female genital mutilation given above.

Description of the different types of female genital mutilation

Female genital mutilation is usually performed by traditional practitioners, generally elderly women in the community specially designated for this task, or traditional birth attendants. In some countries, health professionals—trained midwives and physicians—are increasingly performing female genital mutilation. In Egypt, for example, preliminary results from the 1995 Demographic and Health Survey indicate that the proportion of women who reported having been "circumcised" by a doctor was 13%. In contrast, among their most recently "circumcised" daughters,

1. DEFINITIONS AND CLASSIFICATIONS

46% had been "circumcised" by a doctor. Further aspects of this development are considered in section 5.

The procedures employed in each type of female genital mutilation are described below.

Type I

In the commonest form of this procedure the clitoris is held between the thumb and index finger, pulled out and amputated with one stroke of a sharp object. Bleeding is usually stopped by packing the wound with gauzes or other substances and applying a pressure bandage. Modern trained practitioners may insert one or two stitches around the clitoral artery to stop the bleeding.

Type II

The degree of severity of cutting varies considerably in this type. Commonly the clitoris is amputated as described above and the labia minora are partially or totally removed, often with the same stroke. Bleeding is stopped with packing and bandages or by a few circular stitches which may or may not cover the urethra and part of the vaginal opening. There are reported cases of extensive excisions which heal with fusion of the raw surfaces, resulting in pseudo-infibulation even though there has been no stitching (*24–26*).

Types I and II generally account for 80–85% of all female genital mutilation (*27*), although the proportion may vary greatly from country to country.

Type III

The amount of tissue removed is extensive. The most extreme form involves the complete removal of the clitoris and labia minora, together with the inner surface of the labia majora. The raw edges of the labia majora are brought together to fuse, using thorns, poultices or stitching to hold them in place, and the legs are tied together for 2–6 weeks (*28, 29*). The healed scar creates a "hood of skin" (*17*) which covers the urethra and part or most of the vagina, and which acts as a physical barrier to intercourse. A small opening is left at the back to allow for the flow of urine and menstrual blood. The opening is surrounded by skin and scar tissue and is usually 2–3 cm in diameter but may be as small as the head of a matchstick (*14, 18*).

If after infibulation the posterior opening is large enough, sexual intercourse can take place after gradual dilatation, which may take weeks, months or, in some recorded cases, as long as two years *(21)*. If the opening is too small to start the dilatation, recutting (defibulation) before intercourse is traditionally undertaken by the husband or one of his female relatives using a sharp knife or a piece of glass. Modern couples may seek the assistance of a trained health professional, although this is done in secrecy, possibly because it might "undermine the social image of the man's virility" *(30)*.

In almost all cases of infibulation *(15, 17, 18)* and in many cases of severe excision *(26)*, defibulation must also be performed during childbirth to allow exit of the fetal head without tearing the surrounding scar tissue. If no experienced birth attendant is available to perform defibulation, fetal and/or maternal complications may occur because of obstructed labour or perineal tears.

Traditionally, "re-infibulation" is performed after the woman gives birth. The raw edges are stitched together again to create a small posterior opening, often the same size as that which existed before marriage. This is done to create the illusion of virginity, since a tight vaginal opening is culturally perceived as more pleasurable to the man *(30)*. Because of the extent of both the initial and repeated cutting and suturing, the physical, sexual and psychological effects of infibulation are greater and longer-lasting than for other types of female genital mutilation.

Although only an estimated 15–20% of all women who experience genital mutilation undergo type III, in certain countries such as Djibouti, Somalia and Sudan the proportion is 80–90%. Infibulation is practised on a smaller scale in parts of Egypt, Eritrea, Ethiopia, Gambia, Kenya and Mali, and may occur in other communities where information is lacking or still incomplete.

Type IV

Type IV female genital mutilation encompasses a variety of procedures, most of which are self-explanatory. Two procedures are described here *(13)*.

The term "angurya cuts" describes the scraping of the tissue around the vaginal opening.

"Gishiri cuts" are posterior (or backward) cuts from the vagina into the perineum as an attempt to increase the vaginal outlet to relieve obstructed labour. They often result in vesicovaginal fistulae and damage to the anal sphincter.

2.
Prevalence and epidemiology

Background

Documentation of the prevalence of different types of female genital mutilation began in the early twentieth century with reports by European travellers and missionaries. Since the 1950s, small studies have been undertaken by physicians and gynaecologists in some countries, using clinical records or direct interviews with patients (*15, 16, 31*).

The first national survey ever to be undertaken was conducted by the Faculty of Medicine of the University of Khartoum in Sudan in 1979 (*19*). The Sudan Fertility Survey, also conducted in 1979 (*32*), and the Demographic and Health Survey of Sudan in 1990 (*33*), also included questions on female genital mutilation. Sudan is the only country with comprehensive and reliable national prevalence data over time.

In 1993, the inclusion of a basic module questionnaire on female genital mutilation in the Demographic and Health Surveys[1] was approved (J. Sullivan, Demographic and Health Surveys, personal communication), and has since been used in several countries in Africa. Demographic and Health Survey data on female genital mutilation have recently become available for Central African Republic, Côte d'Ivoire, Egypt, Eritrea, Mali and Yemen. The United Republic of Tanzania has also included questions on female genital mutilation in its current Demographic and Health Survey. It is hoped that if the module is adopted by other countries as well, more accurate data on national prevalence of female genital mutilation will become available.

The first comprehensive article on the epidemiology of female genital mutilation worldwide was published by Hosken in 1978 (*7*). In 1979, the first edition of *The Hosken report* was published, in which the author presented a global review and country-by-country estimates of the prevalence of the practice (*34*). Although the report did not specify the exact

---

[1] The national Demographic and Health Surveys are prepared and organized by Macro International Inc., 11785 Beltville Drive, Calverton, MD 20705, USA.

methodology by which the data were collected, these figures remain a major source for global estimates of female genital mutilation. A literature review of available studies by Toubia published in 1993 (*35*) made modifications to Hosken's figures on the basis of more recent country studies and reports. These figures were updated again in 1995 (*27*) and 1996 (*36*).

Current estimates of prevalence are presented in Table 1 and are based on an extensive review of the most recent published literature and unpublished reports and on the most recent results from completed Demographic and Health Surveys. For countries for which results of studies with adequate sample size or regional representation were available, the estimates are based on such studies. However, the majority of published studies and surveys had sample sizes that were too small, not representative or clinically based. In addition, some reports did not state clearly how the samples were selected. The authors are also aware of a number of other studies, including several Demographic and Health Surveys and a comparative study of the results obtained using the Demographic and Health Survey module in African countries, which are currently under way or whose results became available too late for inclusion. For countries where no specific or reliable studies were found, Hosken's latest estimates are used. On the basis of these figures it is estimated that over 132 million women and girls have experienced female genital mutilation. It is also estimated that some two million girls are at risk of undergoing some form of the procedure every year.

Africa

Benin (estimated prevalence 50%)

A study undertaken by the National Committee on Harmful Traditional Practices in 1993 indicated a prevalence of 50% (*39*). Female genital mutilation is practised mainly in the northern region, in the provinces of Atacora, Borgou and Zou. It is virtually non-existent in the provinces of Atlantic and Mono. The main ethnic groups practising female genital mutilation include the Bariba, Boko, Nago, Peul and Wama. The procedure is most commonly carried out between the ages of 5 and 10, although among the Nago it is often undertaken in adult women after they have already given birth several times. Type II is the most common form reported.

2. PREVALENCE AND EPIDEMIOLOGY

Table 1. Current estimates of female genital mutilation

Country	Female population[a]	Prevalence[b]	Number
Benin	2 730 000	50	1 365 000
Burkina Faso	5 224 000	70	3 656 800
Cameroon	6 684 000	20	1 336 800
Central African Rep.	1 767 000	43	759 810
Chad	3 220 000	60	1 932 000
Côte d'Ivoire	7 089 000	43	3 048 270
Democratic Republic of the Congo	22 158 000	5	1 107 900
Djibouti	254 000	98	248 920
Egypt	28 769 000	97	27 905 930
Eritrea	1 777 000[c]	90	1 599 300
Ethiopia	2 087 000	85	24 723 950
Gambia	496 000	80	396 800
Ghana	8 784 000	30	2 635 200
Guinea	3 333 000	60	1 999 800
Guinea-Bissau	545 000	50	272 500
Kenya	13 935 000	50	6 967 500
Liberia	1 504 000	60	902 400
Mali	5 485 000	94	5 155 900
Mauritania	1 181 000	25	295 250
Niger	4 606 000	20	921 200
Nigeria	64 003 000	40	25 601 200
Senegal	4 190 000	20	838 000
Sierra Leone	2 408 000	90	2 167 200
Somalia	5 137 000	98	5 034 260
Sudan	14 400 000	89	12 816 000
Togo	2 089 000	50	1 044 500
Uganda	10 261 000	5	513 050
United Republic of Tanzania	15 520 000	10	1 552 000
Total			136 797 440

[a] *The world's women.* New York, NY, United Nations, 1995 (*37*).
[b] Prevalence expressed as a percentage. Prevalences for Central African Republic, Côte d'Ivoire, Egypt, Mali and Sudan from Demographic and Health Survey results.
[c] *World population prospects: the 1994 revision.* New York, NY, United Nations, 1994 (*38*).

Burkina Faso (estimated prevalence 70%)

A limited study in 1993 of 805 female genital mutilations indicated prevalence of 73% among girls aged 12–14 years and 88% among women aged 20–24 (*40*). There was little difference between rural and urban areas. However, among girls whose mothers had received secondary education, prevalence was significantly lower (48%) than among those whose mothers had not (78%). Subsequently, the national committee working to control the practice (Comité National de Lutte contre la Pratique de l'Excision) reported that it was widespread among Christians, Muslims and animists in the provinces of Comeo, Ganzourgou, Houet, Kenedougou, Kossi, Kadiogo, Mouhoun, Nahouri, Yatenga and Zounweogo. All groups practise types I and II. The Gourounsi, Leo and Tiebele do not practise female genital mutilation. A limited survey in 1995 showed that prevalence of type I in girls aged 2–3 years was 70.6%. Prevalence of type II in the age group 12–14 was 70.5% and in the age group 20–24 was 80.1% (*41*). This report provides the basis for the current prevalence estimate.

Cameroon (estimated prevalence 20%)

Female genital mutilation is prevalent in certain areas of Cameroon. There are no published studies of national prevalence, but a study by the National Committee on Harmful Traditional Practices in 1994 covered the southwest and far north provinces where the practice is known to occur (*42*). The sample was not stratified and was selected randomly from primary schools, maternity units, traditional birth attendants and communities. In this highly selected population, female genital mutilation was practised by 100% of Muslims and by 63.6% of Christians. Only types I and II were reported. The total prevalence rate for the country, estimated by observers to be 20%, is based on anecdotal evidence.

Central African Republic (estimated prevalence 43%)

The 1994–1995 national Demographic and Health Survey provided the first comprehensive data on female genital mutilation in the country (*43*), indicating an overall prevalence of 43%. However, the rate varies by region and ethnic group. Région Sanitaire IV was found to have the highest prevalence at 91% and, among ethnic groups, prevalence was greatest among the Banda and Mandjia at 84% and 71% respectively. While there was no significant difference between rural and urban dwellers, there was a strong difference between women with no education or with primary schooling (47%) and those with secondary education (23%). There is some indication that prevalence is declining, as it was found to be 53% among women aged 45–49 years and only 35% among women aged 15–19. However, the lower figure in the latter group may be partly due to the fact that nearly 10% of genital mutilations are undertaken after the age of 15, so this age group may include women who have not yet undergone the procedure. In general, however, the majority of girls undergo genital mutilation between the ages of 7 and 15. The survey provided no information on the types practised.

Chad (estimated prevalence 60%)

A UNICEF-supported study was undertaken in the south, east and central regions and in N'Djamena, covering nine communities (unpublished data, 1991). Types I and II were found to predominate; type III was not reported. This partial study is the basis of the current prevalence estimate.

Côte d'Ivoire (estimated prevalence 43%)

The 1994 national Demographic and Health Survey provided the first reliable data (*44*) and indicated an overall prevalence of 43%. This varied from 31% in Abidjan to 57% in the rural savannah region; however, overall prevalence in the rural areas was 45%. Female genital mutilation was found to be much more prevalent among the Muslim population (80%) than among Catholics and Protestants (16%). The most striking difference was between women with no education (55%) and those with primary or secondary education (24%). There does appear to be a slight trend toward reduced prevalence, as the rates for age groups 25–29 and 30–34 were 47% while the rate for those aged 15–19 was 35%. While some women in the latter group may not yet have undergone the procedure, the majority of girls have done so before the age of 10. The survey provided no information on the types of genital mutilation performed.

Democratic Republic of the Congo (estimated prevalence 5%)

No report by a national group or published study was found. The current prevalence estimate is based on previous estimates by Hosken.

Djibouti (estimated prevalence 98%)

There have been no official studies on prevalence in Djibouti, but the Ministry of Health and the national women's union (Union National des Femmes de Djibouti) have reported that female genital mutilation is almost universal, with type III the most common procedure (*45*).

Egypt (estimated prevalence 97%)

The preliminary results of the 1995 national Demographic and Health Survey show a surprisingly higher rate than previously estimated. A validation study is currently being conducted by the Egyptian Fertility Care Society on a subsample, comparing self-reporting and clinical examination. The final results of the survey and the validation study should yield valuable information, as the survey included extensive questions on the procedure, complications, "circumcision" of women's daughters, and attitudes and beliefs.

Female genital mutilation is practised throughout the country by Muslims and Christians. Type I is the common procedure, although type III is reported in areas of south Egypt closer to Sudan (*46, 47*).

Eritrea (estimated prevalence 90%)

In 1993, Eritrea gained independence from Ethiopia. Female genital mutilation is known to be practised by Eritrean Christians and Muslims. The Eritrean People's Liberation Front, which is the governing party, and the National Union of Eritrean Women, have taken a position against the practice since the 1970s. There are no published statistics on prevalence in Eritrea following independence from Ethiopia. While two surveys conducted in Ethiopia in 1985 and 1990 (see section on Ethiopia, below) did not produce statistics specific to Eritrea, which was a war zone at the time, they give the general impression that female genital mutilation is as widespread in Eritrea as it is in Ethiopia. Results from the recent Demographic and Health Survey in Eritrea will provide the first reliable data on prevalence.

Ethiopia (estimated prevalence 85%)

Female genital mutilation is common among Christians and Muslims, and was practised by Ethiopian Jews, who now live in Israel. Types I and II are common except in the areas bordering Somalia, particularly Hararghe, where type III is practised. In 1984, the Ethiopian Ministry of Health together with UNICEF conducted a prevalence survey in five regions — Addis Ababa, Arssi, Eritrea, Gojjam and Hararghe (*48*). The findings suggest that the practice is almost universal in the areas studied, although no overall prevalence rates are cited. A further survey in 1990, sponsored by IAC, included 20 of the 31 administrative regions, covering 73% of the population of the country (*49*). This showed that 85% of the women surveyed had undergone genital mutilation. There is some regional overlap between the two surveys. However, high prevalence regions such as Diredawa, Eastern Hararghe and Ogaden were not included in the 1990 survey. Two ethnic groups, the Begas and the Wellega, do not practise female genital mutilation.

Gambia (estimated prevalence 80%)

A study by Singhateh published in 1985, covering several regions in Gambia, indicated a prevalence rate of 79% (*50*). However, the sample was not representative of the total population. The study reported different prevalence rates for different ethnic groups (100% for the Mandinga and Serehule, 93% for the Fula, 65.7% for the Jola and only 1.9% for the Wollof). All groups practise types I and II.

Ghana (estimated prevalence 30%)

According to Kadri (*51*), female genital mutilation is practised in two secluded regions of Ghana — in the Upper East region by the Bussansi, Frafra, Kantonsi, Kassena, Kussasi, Mamprushie, Moshie and Nankanne ethnic groups and in the Upper West region by the Dargarti, Grunshie, Kantonsi, Lobi, Sissala and Walas ethnic groups. Adherence to the practice in these regions ranges from 75% to 100%. A study by Twumasi (*52*) in Accra and Nsawam in the south found female genital mutilation only among migrant communities from the northern part of Ghana and from neighbouring countries.

Guinea (estimated prevalence 60%)

No studies have been conducted on prevalence and estimates are based on reporting by the National Committee on Harmful Traditional Practices (Cellule de Coordination sur les Pratiques Traditionnelles Affectant la Femme et l'Enfant, CPTAFE; unpublished data, 1991).

Guinea-Bissau (estimated prevalence 50%)

A limited non-representative survey by the national women's union (Union Démocratique des Femmes de la Guinée-Bissau) reported type II female genital mutilation in almost 100% of Muslim women (unpublished data, 1990). Muslims constitute about 50% of the population.

Kenya (estimated prevalence 50%)

Types I, II and III have all been reported in Kenya, where they are practised by several ethnic groups. The Maendeleo ya Wanawake Organization, the largest women's organization in Kenya, conducted a survey in 1991 in four districts in which female genital mutilation is known to be widely practised — Kisii, Meru, Narok and Samburu (*53*). The overall prevalence in these districts was 89.6%. There are no surveys of other districts in Kenya. Given that female genital mutilation is not practised in some major districts and that it is being abandoned by the increasing urban population, prevalence is currently estimated at 50% for the country as a whole.

Liberia (estimated prevalence 60%)

According to a 1984 report (54), female genital mutilation is practised in most parts of Liberia and only three ethnic groups do not perform it. The estimated prevalence, based on a limited survey, is between 50% and 70%. The practice, type II only, is part of the initiation into the secret Sande or bush school.

Mali (estimated prevalence 94%)

The results from the 1995–1996 national Demographic and Health Survey indicate an overall prevalence of 94% (55). Female genital mutilation is practised throughout Mali, except for the regions of Gao and Tombouktou. Types I and II are predominant (52% and 47% respectively), with type III representing less than 1%. There are no significant differences in prevalence between women from rural areas and those from urban areas, or between women with no education or primary education (94%) and those with secondary education (90%). Female genital mutilation is practised by all religious groups, ranging from 85% among Christians to 94% among Muslims, and across all ethnic groups. The two groups with lower prevalence rates are the Tamacheck (16%) and the Sonrai (48%), both of which reside mainly in the regions of Gao and Tombouktou.

Mauritania (estimated prevalence 25%)

According to the Director of Social Affairs in the Ministry of Health of Mauritania, 20–25% of the population undergo female genital mutilation (unpublished data, 1987).

Niger (estimated prevalence 20%)

While there are no published studies on national prevalence, two published reports indicate that female genital mutilation is practised in three provinces: Diffa, Niamey and Tillabery (56, 57). The ethnic groups concerned who perform mainly types I and II are the Arabes (Shuwa), Gourmanche, Kourtey, Peulh, Songhai and Wogo. These reports from 1992 and 1993 are the basis of the current prevalence estimate.

Nigeria (estimated prevalence 40%)

Female genital mutilation is acknowledged to be widely practised in Nigeria and particularly among the three major tribes — the Hausa, Ibo and Yoruba. The practice is said to be declining in large urban centres. In 1985, the Nigerian Association of Nurses and Nurse-midwives conducted a national but non-representative survey and found that 13 out of 21 states had populations who practise female genital mutilation (*58*). Types I, II and III were all reported, as were gishiri cuts (type IV). Based on this limited sample, the average prevalence for the areas surveyed was 39.2%. This is considered low by many observers given that major ethnic groups practise female genital mutilation.

Senegal (estimated prevalence 20%)

A national study by Mottin-Sylla (*59*) reported prevalence in 1990 at around 18%, revising the 1976 estimate of 35%.

Sierra Leone (estimated prevalence 90%)

According to a 1984 study by Koso-Thomas (*20*), all Christian and Muslim ethnic groups in the country practise female genital mutilation, except for the Krios who live in the western region and in the capital of Freetown. Only types I and II are performed as part of the initiation rituals of the Bundo and Sande secret societies. The current prevalence estimate is based on the reporting by Koso-Thomas.

Somalia (estimated prevalence 98%)

Two documents published in 1982 and 1989 indicate that female genital mutilation is almost universal in Somalia with over 80% of procedures being of type III and the remainder type I (*60, 61*).

Sudan (estimated prevalence 89%)

The 1990 Sudan Demographic and Health Survey reported that 89% of ever-married women in the northern, eastern and western provinces had been "circumcised" (*33*). This is a 7% drop from the 96% found in the Sudan Fertility Survey of 1979 (*32*). The majority of women (85%) had undergone type III and only 15% had undergone type I. There was little variation in the distribution of types of female genital mutilation between rural and urban areas but there were differences in type by region. Twice as many women under 25 years (20%) as those over 40 years (10%) had undergone type I. Female genital mutilation is not practised in the three southern provinces of Sudan.

Togo *(estimated prevalence 50%)*

The National Committee on Harmful Traditional Practices has reported that female genital mutilation is common in the region of Tchaoudjo in the north (unpublished data). No national surveys or studies have been reported. The current prevalence estimate is based on the committee's report.

Uganda *(estimated prevalence 5%)*

There are no published studies on prevalence. The figure of 5% has been derived from anecdotal evidence which gives the general impression that prevalence is very low, with only one or two tribes practising female genital mutilation. A video produced by IAC in 1993 shows the genital mutilation of young women over 16 years of age during a village ceremony in Uganda, but does not comment on the overall prevalence or ethnic distribution of the practice (*62*).

United Republic of Tanzania *(estimated prevalence 10%)*

Types I and II are reported in the Arusha, Dodoma, Iringa, Kiliminjaro, Mara, Ngorogoro and Singida regions (*63*). In some groups, such as the Shaga of Mount Kilimanjaro, prevalence is high. Infibulation (type III) is performed by Somali settlers and refugees. The current national estimate is based on IAC reports and could be an underestimate. Results from the national Demographic and Health Survey will provide the first comprehensive prevalence data.

Refugee and immigrant populations

The presence of increasing numbers of refugees and immigrants from countries where female genital mutilation is practised in Australia, Europe, and North America has aroused much interest in this issue in the host countries. As a result several countries have passed laws against female genital mutilation even though little is known about the numbers and characteristics of African communities in these countries. In some countries, programmes have been started to reach out to the community or to alert health and social services to protect girls at risk of genital mutilation.

2. PREVALENCE AND EPIDEMIOLOGY

Australia

The Government of Australia is supporting a national education programme on female genital mutilation (1995–2000) directed at relevant communities and health and welfare professionals. The draft operating framework for the programme (Department of Human Services, 1996) states that:

"Recent migration patterns to Australia indicate an increase in the numbers of people now living in Australia from countries where female genital mutilation is traditionally practised. According to the 1991 Australian Bureau of Statistics Census, there were approximately 76,000 women living in Australia from countries where some form of female genital mutilation is practised. Current estimates are that more than 87,000 women and girls are now living in Australia from these countries."

Europe

There are significant numbers of Somalis and smaller numbers of other African refugees and immigrants in Denmark, Netherlands, Norway and Sweden. There are no reports on the exact numbers of these populations.

There are large numbers of immigrants in France from several West African countries. A women's group for the abolition of female genital mutilation (Groupes femmes pour l'abolition des mutilations sexuelles, GAMS) has reported that there are at least 27 000 women and girls with genital mutilation in France (unpublished data, 1992).

Italy has a large population of Ethiopian, Eritrean and Somali immigrants. However, there are no reports on the exact numbers of these groups.

The United Kingdom of Great Britain and Northern Ireland has a large number of immigrants and refugees from Egypt, Eritrea, Ethiopia, Ghana, Nigeria, Somalia and Sudan, and smaller numbers from other African countries. In Britain the Labour Force Survey (1988) estimated the settled African population in Britain was 122 000, representing an increase of 30% since 1981. Since 1988, the number of African nationals coming to the United Kingdom has doubled to around 8000 per year. The largest proportion of these are refugees from the Horn of Africa. The Foundation for Women's Health, Research and Development (FORWARD) has assisted the Department of Health and local authorities in developing a culturally sensitive policy and education programmes on female genital mutilation targeted at the communities concerned.

In 1991, FORWARD conducted a survey (funded by the Department of Health and approved by the Association of Directors of Social Services) to assess the level of casework intervention within local authorities.

Of the 65 local social work departments canvassed, 10 reported casework intervention because of suspected female genital mutilation (*64*). The Department of Health is sponsoring FORWARD to map out the profiles of communities for whom female genital mutilation is a deep-rooted traditional practice and to review all the programmes implemented to date on female genital mutilation in the United Kingdom. The outcome of this project will be published.

North America

The African Resource Centre in Ottawa, Canada, has reported 12 000 African immigrants in the city but did not indicate whether they came from countries where female genital mutilation is practised (unpublished data, 1993). Canada receives immigrants and refugees from all over Africa but the numbers of Eritreans, Ethiopians and Somalis have increased significantly in the past 10 years.

The United States of America receives immigrants and refugees from all African countries. The 1990 census, which does not carry detailed information on the country of origin of citizens and residents, indicated that the total African-born population was 363 819 and that 10 357 African-born immigrants were admitted to the country between 1991 and 1994. According to preliminary statistics collected by the Research, Action and Information Network for Bodily Integrity of Women (RAINB♀), women constitute 40.7% of the African-born population in the country. The 11 largest groups come from the following countries: Egypt, Ethiopia, Ghana, Kenya, Liberia, Nigeria, Sierra Leone, Somalia, Sudan, Uganda and the United Republic of Tanzania. The prevalence of female genital mutilation varies widely among populations from these countries. RAINB♀ is currently undertaking a study of African immigrants in the New York metropolitan area, *inter alia* collecting population statistics and conducting a needs assessment for health and social services. The aim of this study is to assist women who have suffered from genital mutilation and to prevent its occurrence among immigrant children.

Israel

Between 1984 and 1990, the Government of Israel undertook a major resettlement programme for the entire Jewish population of Ethiopia. This group is known to practise female genital mutilation (*65*). A preliminary report (*66*) did not find evidence of a continuation of the practice following immigration but a more thorough investigation is needed to substantiate this. A recent study by Asali et al. (*67*), which included interviews with 21 Bedouin women, indicated that female genital mutilation has been practised in this ethnic group. Girls are most commonly "circumcised" between the ages of 12 and 17. However, physical examination of 37 young women from these tribes revealed only small scars on the prepuce of the clitoris or on the upper labia minora, indicating that the procedure may have been modified to a non-cutting ritual in more recent years.

Evidence of prevalence in other regions

Arabian peninsula

A limited inquiry on female genital mutilation conducted in the city of Sana'a, Yemen (S. Thadeus, unpublished data, 1992), found that the practice was localized to a few ethnic groups, and was predominantly of type I. The primary groups involved had historically been traders across the Red Sea and some had settled in East Africa. The recent national Demographic and Health Survey included two questions on female genital mutilation. These questions did not refer to prevalence in Yemen, but asked whether women approved or disapproved of the practice and what their reasons were for approval or disapproval.

Bahrain, Oman, Saudi Arabia and United Arab Emirates are listed in some publications as having female genital mutilation. No national reports or documented evidence were found regarding the practice in these countries.

South and South-East Asia

According to reports by Ghadially (68) and Srinivasan (69), female genital mutilation is practised in India by the small ethno-religious minority, the Daudi Bohra of the Ismaili Shia sect of Islam. The total population concerned is around half a million in the Bombay area and in small immigrant communities in Africa and North America.

According to Pratiknya of Gadjah Mada University in Indonesia, genital cutting operations took place in that country in the past but are no longer performed in the country (70). However, various non-cutting rituals involving the clitoris still persist in Indonesia. These include cleaning with herbal juice, symbolic cutting and light puncture of the clitoris. According to the 1997 WHO/UNICEF/UNFPA classification, symbolic cutting and light puncture of the clitoris are considered to be type IV female genital mutilation.

Several writers have reported genital mutilation practices among some Muslims in Malaysia but no reports by national groups or documented evidence of the practice have been found.

Latin America

Several authors have mentioned the practice of female genital mutilation among indigenous people in Colombia, Mexico and Peru. No reports from national organizations or published studies were found. In the city of São Paulo in Brazil, a newspaper claimed that female genital mutilation is being practised among Egyptian immigrant communities. Further investigation revealed no documented evidence of such practices.

3.
Health consequences

Development and functional anatomy of the external female genitalia

To understand fully the health consequences of the different types of female genital mutilation and, particularly, the difference between male circumcision and female genital mutilation, it is important to have a basic understanding of the development and functional anatomy of the female genitals. This section also provides a brief description of the contribution of the normal genitals to the sexual response in women.

The embryological origins and the functional anatomy of the primary external genitalia of the male (the penis) and the female (the clitoris and labia minora) are very similar. According to Gilbert (71):

> "At the end of the embryonic period the external genitalia of the male and the female are similar in appearance, but during the third month the genital tubercle in the male becomes a recognizable penis and the labioscrotal swellings fuse to form the scrotum ... In the female the genital tubercle becomes the clitoris. The urogenital folds remain unfused and become the labia minora, while the labioscrotal swellings become the labia majora."

Stilwell (72) compared the anatomy of the genitalia of human males and females as follows:

> "Many parts of the vulva are comparable or specifically homologous to male organs, but have adapted to vagina and vulva as a receptacle and canal for parturition. For example, the vestibular bulbs (male corpus spongiosum) are divided to flank the vagina, thus, do not enclose the urethra. Vascular and nervous structures are comparable: the pudendal nerve and the internal pudendal vessels, pelvic splanchnic and hypogastric nerve plexus".

The external female genitalia lie within the vulva and comprise the clitoris (equivalent to the tip of the penis and end of the shaft), the labia minora (equivalent to the shaft of the penis), the labia majora (equivalent to the scrotum), and the opening to the vagina.

The clitoris has four distinct parts: a small glans or head, a short body of two incompletely separated corpora cavernosa, continuous posteriorly with a pair of crura (72). All the parts are made of spongy, vascular, erectile tissue. The mature clitoris (glans and body) is about 2–2.5 cm in length with the crura twice as long. The size varies widely between individuals, depending on genetic and endocrine influence. Its prominence outside the lips varies with the development of the adjacent vulva.

The prepuce (foreskin) is a fold of epithelium above the clitoris which may or may not cover the entire glans. In young girls it is not well developed (2–3 mm in length) and difficult to separate from the glans. This is important to remember when comparing type I female genital mutilation to male circumcision.

The labia majora are two prominent longitudinal cutaneous (skin) folds extending from the mons veneris to the anterior boundary of the perineum. Their outer surface is pigmented and covered with hair and the inner surface is smooth and contains large sebaceous (lubricating) follicles.

The labia minora are made of cavernous erectile tissue with a high concentration of sensory nerve endings.

Lowry (73) summarizes the histological evidence regarding the sensitivity of the female external genitalia as follows:

"In summary, the clitoris contains, in most women, a large number of receptor nerve endings; in some women, other areas may contain more. In almost all women, the labia minora are also highly sensitive."

The vagina is the least sensitive area, with sensory nerve endings limited to a ring around the inlet.

The above descriptions indicate the importance of the clitoris and labia minora as the primary sensory organs in the female sexual response. Cutting part or all of them will undoubtedly interfere with, though not necessarily abolish, the physical receptivity of sexual stimulation in women. Human sexual arousal is also brought about by other sensory and non-sensory stimulants. The secondary organs include the lips, breasts and other areas of heightened sexual sensitivity. Non-tactile physical senses, such as smell, vision and hearing, can transmit sexually stimulating messages. Individuals vary in terms of their psychological predisposition towards sexual arousal as well as in their ability to achieve sexual satisfaction. Emotions, as part of the psychological milieux within which sexual arousal occurs, are known to be a strong factor, particularly in women. Finally, social conditioning with regard to appropriate sexual behaviour plays a crucial role in both sexual arousal and the ability to seek and attain sexual pleasure. The impact of female genital mutilation on sexual response is discussed in more detail below.

Physical consequences and complications

All types of female genital mutilation involve removal or damage to the normal functioning of the external female genitalia and can give rise to a range of well documented physical complications. Psychological effects are less well documented in the scientific literature but descriptions are abundant in anecdotal evidence and in women's stories of their experiences (74).

The occurrence of physical complications depends on several factors, including the extent of cutting, the skill of the operator, the cleanliness of the tools used on the surrounding area, and the physical condition of the child. Although serious complications are possible following all types of female genital mutilation, those resulting from type III occur more frequently, tend to be more serious and last longer. Complications may be fewer when the procedure is undertaken by a skilled operator, although cases of death from uncontrolled bleeding from the clitoral artery have occurred even when it was performed by a trained physician (75).

The physical complications listed below are summarized from the published literature and focus on the short-term and long-term problems that occur with types I, II and III.

Immediate complications — all types

Death

While anecdotal evidence is frequently mentioned (18, 21), no study has ever been undertaken to determine the proportion of female child mortality that is attributable to female genital mutilation. Death can result from severe bleeding (haemorrhagic shock), from the pain and trauma (neurogenic shock) or from severe and overwhelming infection (septicaemia). Asuen reported a case of a 23-year-old multiparous Nigerian woman who was "circumcised" one day prior to admission for delivery. A live baby girl was delivered but the woman's circumcision wound became infected and four days later she became comatose and died (76).

Haemorrhage

Severe bleeding (haemorrhage) is the most common immediate complication and evidence of its high incidence is abundant in the literature (18, 21, 77). In El Dareer's study, bleeding accounted for almost one-quarter (22%) of all reported complications (19, 78). Amputation of the clitoris cuts across the clitoral artery in which blood flows at high pressure. To stop the bleeding, the artery must be packed tightly or tied with a running stitch, either of which may slip and lead to haemorrhage (*79*). Secondary haemorrhage can occur after the first week as a result of sloughing of the clot over the artery owing to infection. An acute episode of haemorrhage or protracted bleeding can lead to anaemia (*80*) or, if very severe, to death.

Shock

Immediately after the procedure the child may enter a state of shock from the pain, psychological trauma and exhaustion from screaming. The short-term and long-term effects of this state of physical and psychological shock have not been reported.

Injury to neighbouring organs

As the procedure is commonly performed with no anaesthesia or with local anaesthesia only, the girl screams and wriggles from fear and pain. The cutting instrument may be crude and the practitioner may be inexperienced or have failing eyesight. Any of these can result in injury to the urethra (*18*), the vagina, the perineum or the rectum and can lead to the formation of fistulae through which urine or faeces will leak continuously (*81*).

Urine retention

Pain, swelling and inflammation around the wound and subsequent infection can lead to urine retention, which may last for hours or days, but is usually reversible. Intervention with a catheter or removal of stitches may be necessary before urine can be passed normally.

Infection

Infection is very common and can be caused by unsterile instruments. It can also occur within a few days of the operation as the area becomes soaked in urine and contaminated by faeces (*21*). The degree of infection varies widely from a superficial wound infection to a generalized blood infection or septicaemia. Unsterilized tools and faecal matter can cause infection with tetanus spores or bacteria that will cause gangrene.

Severe pain

The majority of procedures are performed without anaesthetic. When local anaesthesia is used, pain in the highly sensitive area of the clitoris returns within 2–3 hours of the operation. Applying the local anaesthesia is itself extremely painful because the area of the clitoris and labia minora has a dense concentration of nerves and is highly sensitive. The use of general anaesthesia adds to the risk of death since it is usually not applied by a specialist with paediatric experience.

Long-term complications of types I and II

Failure to heal

Infection, separation by the urine flow and movement during walking may prevent the wound edges from healing. A weeping wound oozing pus or a chronic infected ulcer may result, which will require proper dressing and expert handling. Even if healing is complete, the rigid vulnerable scar over the clitoris may split open during childbirth. This may lead to renewed profuse bleeding from the clitoral artery.

Abscess formation

In cases where the infection is buried under the wound edges or an embedded stitch fails to be absorbed, an abscess can form which will usually require surgical incision and repeated dressing over a period of time.

Dermoid cyst

This is the most common long-term complication of all types of female genital mutilation. It results from the embedding of skin tissue in the scar. The gland which normally lubricates the skin will continue to secrete under the scar and form a cyst or sac full of cheesy material. The reported size of dermoid cysts ranges from that of a small pea to that of a grapefruit or football. Although not a serious threat to physical health these cysts are extremely distressing (*82*). Small dermoid cysts should be left alone to avoid further damage to the area, and the woman should be reassured. If cysts become very large or infected, surgical removal may be unavoidable.

Keloids

There is a genetic susceptibility to keloids (excessive growth of scar tissue) in many of the ethnic groups that practice female genital mutilation. Vulval keloids are disfiguring and psychologically distressing. Treatment is often unsuccessful since surgical removal frequently provokes further growth.

Urinary tract infection

Presence of pus and infection near the short urethra can cause recurrent ascending urinary tract infections.

Scar neuroma

Trapping of the clitoral nerve in a stitch or in the scar tissue of the healed wound can result in a neuroma (tumour consisting of neural tissue). This can make touching the vulva during sexual intercourse or during washing very painful.

Painful sexual intercourse

Sexual intercourse can become painful and psychologically distressing as a result of one or several of the complications mentioned above.

HIV/AIDS, hepatitis B and other bloodborne diseases

Although female genital mutilation may increase an individual's risk of acquiring bloodborne pathogens such as the human immunodeficiency virus (HIV) or the hepatitis B virus there is, as yet, no evidence that it is a major contributor to the spread of the acquired immunodeficiency syndrome (AIDS) (83), hepatitis B or other bloodborne diseases. However, a recent study in Kenya reported that group operations, using the same unclean cutting instruments, with consequent risk of transmission, are still common (53).

Pseudo-infibulation

Excessive type II female genital mutilation can heal with vulval adhesions (23) creating a pseudo-infibulation even when there is no stitching of the labia .

Long-term complications of type III

As cutting is more extensive in type III female genital mutilation, the long-term complications include those mentioned for types I and II along with those listed below. Additional complications are possible as a result of mechanical obstruction caused by the scarring covering the urethra and vagina, and the further damage caused by defibulation and by "re-infibulation".

Reproductive tract infections

Ascending infections from the vulva due to retained discharge and blood can lead to pelvic inflammatory disease (*84*). The rate of pelvic inflammatory disease in infibulated women is three times that in women with clitoridectomy only. The rate of pelvic inflammatory disease in women who have undergone clitoridectomy is often higher than that in women who have not undergone genital mutilation (*15*). The possible causes are infection at the time of the operation, interference in the drainage of urine and vaginal secretions, and postpartum wound infection. Pelvic inflammatory disease is not only painful but can also lead to infertility as a result of scarring of the fallopian tubes. The contribution of infibulation to the high levels of infertility in Africa is contested — some studies claim a high contribution (*29*), but the evidence has been challenged.

Dysmenorrhoea

There are reports of increased dysmenorrhoea (painful menstruation) (*85*), although these have not been verified and possible mechanisms have not been explored. One suggestion is that infection causes increased pelvic congestion. There may also be a psychosomatic element because of increased anxiety over the state of the genitals.

Chronic urinary tract obstruction

A tight infibulation or urethral stricture resulting from accidental injury can cause obstruction of urethral flow, repeated infections and bladder stones.

Urinary incontinence

Dribbling of urine is common in infibulated women; the bladder is not completely emptied and chronic infection under the hood of scar tissue makes control of urine difficult (*21, 86*).

HIV/AIDS, hepatitis B and other bloodborne diseases

Repeated cutting and stitching during labour, higher incidence of wounds and abrasions during sexual intercourse, and the possibility of anal intercourse when vaginal penetration is impossible or difficult may increase the risk of transmission of HIV (*30*), hepatitis B or other bloodborne diseases. Although these are all valid hypotheses, there is no published evidence of any such increase.

Stenosis of the artificial opening to the vagina

With infibulation, the artificial opening to the vagina can be so small that it closes almost completely over time. This may cause incomplete voiding of urine or haematocolpos (retained menstrual blood) and make sexual intercourse impossible (*21*). Products of miscarriage could also be retained in the vaginal canal leading to severe infection. A case of a primary stone in the vagina due to obstruction in a 33-year-old woman from the Ibo ethnic group in Nigeria has been reported (*87*). The stone caused severe pain, infertility and dribbling of urine. Although the Ibo are known to practise type II genital mutilation, in this case the vaginal opening was narrowed by fused labia which created an infibulation-like occlusion.

Complications of labour and delivery

During childbirth, the infibulated woman must be defibulated to allow the fetal head to emerge from the vagina. This increases the risk of bleeding and wound infection. If an experienced attendant is not available to perform defibulation (anterior episiotomy), labour may become obstructed (*88*). Prolonged obstructed labour can cause moderate-to-severe complications for the mother and the child. No studies have been undertaken on the precise impact of infibulation on perinatal outcome. However, cases of ruptured vulval scar, perineal tears, fetal distress and vesicovaginal and vesicorectal fistulae have been reported (*81*). There have also been reports of severe lacerations, including third-degree tears involving the anal musculature and injuries to the urinary tract including avulsion (tearing away) of the urethra from the bladder (*89*). Although female genital mutilation may contribute to maternal mortality there is no evidence of the extent of that contribution. It has been claimed that female genital mutilation doubles the rate of maternal mortality (*90*). This allegation has not been substantiated by any published study. One well documented study was undertaken by DeSilva on 173 mostly infibulated Sudanese women living in Saudi Arabia and delivering in a well-equipped hospital (*88*). There was significant delay in the second stage of labour, increased haemorrhage and increased occurrence of severe fetal asphyxia. There was no increase in maternal or neonatal mortality, which may be the result of the availability of resuscitation facilities in the hospital. Similar effects on labour occurring in rural areas may yield different outcomes. Evidence from Somalia (*77*) regarding the effect of infibulation on fetal and maternal outcome is weak because of small sample size, absence of information on other characteristics of the mothers and no control group. Moreover, the high rates of vesicovaginal and vesicorectal fistulae in Africa occur primarily as a result of pregnancy in very young girls whose pelvises are not well developed. The true contribution of female genital mutilation to this condition has still not been verified.

Injury to neighbouring organs

This can occur during defibulation performed crudely to enable sexual intercourse to take place or during labour. Spontaneous injury or tearing of the perineum can also occur as a result of strong uterine contractions during labour (*81*).

Psychological and sexual effects

The few studies and reports available on the psychological and sexual effects of female genital mutilation are qualitative, in the form of case studies, rather than quantitative in nature, and therefore do not indicate the prevalence of such complications.

Effect on the psychological health of girls

There is only one published case of psychopathology in a child resulting from "fear of circumcision" in the medical literature (*91*).[1] This scarcity probably reflects the lack of attention by the research community to documenting these problems rather than the rarity of the condition. Other evidence suggests that the perception of the incident by the girl is not simply negative, despite the pain and trauma. The desirability of the ceremony for the child, with its social advantages of peer acceptance, personal pride and material gifts is strongly juxtaposed to the physical suffering in the stories of many women (*77, 92*). One description of the opposing forces acting on the child is provided from Burkina Faso (*25*):

> "In areas where excision is practised, unexcised girls are constantly mocked by friends who have undergone the operation. Those yet to be excised may be terrified by older girls' description of what is in store for them."

The balance between the positive and the negative in the girl's experience is what will shape her reaction and will determine how she remembers the incident. A study in Somalia asked 159 girls aged 8–16 to draw their experience of the moment of their "circumcision" and the period of convalescence afterwards (*93*). All the girls remembered the exact day and time they were "circumcised", their age, who the "circumciser" was and where the procedure took place. Psychological analysis of the girls'

---

[1] This study also documented two cases of psychopathology directly related to female genital mutilation in adult women.

drawings indicated that self-esteem and self-identity of the subjects appeared to be disturbed both on the physical and psychological levels. The researchers also found that "circumcision" was not experienced as an event limited in time and then forgotten, but as a factor which remained, even latently, in a girl's thoughts. They concluded that:

> "The circumcision is also considered as an obligatory step towards the conquest of a social identity by the Somali women in order to avoid being an outcast. When, at the conscious level however, this censorship of the unpleasant aspects of the practice and its negative consequences does not come about, even the comments become explosive, and together with the graphic message, indicative of experiences of suffering, devaluation and impotence. It is interesting to note the fact that such data is not influenced by the different forms or the age at which circumcision takes place. Only as the child grows older do the verbal indications of the logistical and socio-cultural aspects of the event increase, in harmony with the intellectual development of the subject. There is also a higher valorisation of the circumcised subject as if age brought about a higher social compensation. Nevertheless, the aspects of anxiety and aggressiveness linked with the event do not subside with age (even over a period of time)."

As more women from different societies feel free to speak about their experiences of genital mutilation, the cumulative evidence suggests that the event is mostly remembered as extremely traumatic and leaves a lifelong emotional scar (50, 92, 94, 95).

Apart from the direct trauma and its possible effects on the psychological health of the girl and her future sexual experience, a more subtle process affects the self-perception of the young girl and shapes her self-esteem. Boddy describes this process after observing the life of women in Hofriyat village of northern Sudan (96):

> "In Hofriyat, I suggest, we need to contemplate the implications of pharonic circumcision for a female child's developing self-perception. Through this operation and other procedures involving pain or trauma, appropriate feminine dispositions are being inculcated in young girls, dispositions which ... are inscribed in their bodies not only physically, but also cognitively and emotionally, in the form of mental inclinations, "schemes of perception and thought." But alone the trauma of pharonic circumcision is insufficient to shape the feminine self, to propel it in culturally prescribed directions: such acts must also be meaningful to those who undergo and reproduce them. Here, as will be seen, meaning is carefully built up through the use of metaphors and associations which combine to establish an identification of circum-

cised women with morally appropriate fertility, hence to orient them toward their all-important generative and transformative roles in Hofriyat society. Paradoxically, however, to achieve this gender identity, women implicitly repudiate their sexuality."

Although female genital mutilation rituals and the symbols and messages which surround them vary between communities, pain and trauma are central in defining appropriate feminine disposition, and concepts of "morally appropriate fertility" and "repudiation of sexuality to achieve socially prescribed gender identity" are common modes of social conditioning of women. In this context, women's sexuality is affected just as much by the processes of social conditioning that accompany genital mutilation as the trauma of the cutting and the physical damage that results from it.

Furthermore, the state of their mutilation becomes such a part of women's bodily image that any alteration to that state threatens their sense of security. A Somali mother of three was advised to stay defibulated to cure the persistent gonorrhoea that had afflicted her and her husband. She acted against medical advice and was "re-infibulated" — her wound became infected and she could hardly walk because of the pain. She did not do this for her husband's gratification but because of her own sense of impurity and shame if she was not "closed" (30). Such are the reasons why women perpetuate the practice and insist that it is done to their daughters. They want to pass on to them the most intimate aspects of their self-perception and feelings of gender and therefore social identity.[1]

Effect on women's sexuality

There are few studies available on the effect of different types of female genital mutilation on the sexuality of adult women. None of these studies attempt to differentiate between the physical and psychological causes of altered sexual response in some genitally-mutilated women and why some women with a particular type of mutilation may experience sexual pleasure while others do not.

Megafu investigated the effect of female genital mutilation on the age at first sexual intercourse and the incidence of premarital coitus among

---

[1] The WHO Human Reproduction Advisory Panel has defined "gender" as the term used to describe those characteristics of men and women which are socially constructed, in contrast to those which are biologically determined. People are born female or male, but learn to be girls and boys who grow into women and men. They are taught what the appropriate behaviour, attitudes, roles and activities are for them. This learned behaviour is what makes up gender identity and determines gender roles.

young Ibo women in Nigeria (*97*). He found no difference in what he termed "levels of promiscuity" between "circumcised" (type II) and "uncircumcised" women. He also reported that only 58.8% of the former experienced orgasm in contrast to 68.7% of the latter. This study also showed that when the clitoris is removed the labia minora and the breasts take over as the most erotic organs in the body.

Shandall studied 4024 women from his outpatient clinic in northern Sudan and reported that over 80% of those with type III (infibulation) did not know of or experience orgasm, compared to around 10% of those with type I or who were "uncircumcised" (*15*). El Dareer conducted a national survey, also in north Sudan, and reported similar results (*19*). In her study, 50% of women reported no sexual pleasure, 23% were indifferent to sexual intercourse and the remainder experienced pleasure all or some of the time. It is important to remember that in northern Sudan over 90% of women undergo type III genital mutilation. Another study, by Lightfoot-Klein, contradicted this evidence; out of 300 Sudanese women with infibulation, 90% reported pleasurable sex with frequent orgasm (*95*). The author does not adequately describe her methodology but admits to using two senior nurses, both with a thriving "circumcision" practice on the side, as her translators. In fact this study contradicts the findings of a previous study by the same author which reported severe pain and suffering with sexual intercourse and lack of pleasure with sex by infibulated women in Sudan (*98*).

Karim and Ammar studied 331 "circumcised" women who attended their outpatient clinic in Cairo (*99*). Of these, 29% did not experience any sexual satisfaction during intercourse, 30% experienced some satisfaction but did not reach orgasm and 41% experienced satisfaction and orgasm frequently. Although the sample contained women with types I, II and III genital mutilation, no clear conclusion was reached as to the difference in sexual experience of women with the different types. Also given possible confounding variables, such as social conditioning and the quality of the marital relationship, these numbers could be meaningful only if compared to the experiences of women with no genital mutilation in the same society. Another study of Egyptian women (133 who had undergone types I and II female genital mutilation and 26 who were "uncircumcised") was conducted by Badawi who reported that a greater proportion of the latter had sexual excitement in response to stimulation of the genitals compared to those with genital mutilation (*100*). The study also found that 50% of the "uncircumcised" women and 25% of those with genital mutilation experienced orgasm with manual stimulation of the clitoris/clitoral area. However, the size of the sample of uncircumcised women was very small.

Koso-Thomas reported on the experience of arousal, sexual feelings from genital stimulation and possibility of reaching climax among "circumcised" women in Sierra Leone (20). Her sample included 47 women with clitoridectomy (type I) and 93 women with clitoridectomy and excision of labia (type II). An interesting finding was the difference between 14 women with sexual experience before the procedure and 33 who experienced sex only afterwards. All respondents were fully conscious of themselves as sexual beings, a perception that the experience of genital mutilation did not seem to alter. With regard to their response to male sexual advances, those who had experienced sex before had positive reactions and those who experienced it only afterwards had a neutral response. When asked about the level of arousal experienced, no woman in either group reported intense arousal but those with previous experience were better able to detect a mild stimulation. None of the women experienced orgasm, but the women with no previous sexual experience remained neutral while those with previous experience became aroused but unfulfilled.

From Burkina Faso, Kere and Tapsoba reported on the sexual experience of several women and men whom they interviewed and who live with the consequences of female genital mutilation (26). Many of the women reported pain and discomfort with intercourse; some experienced a degree of sexual arousal but most did not experience orgasm.

From the evidence cited, it is clear that all types of female genital mutilation interfere to some degree with women's sexual response but do not necessarily abolish the possibility of sexual pleasure and climax. As explained on page 24, some of the sensitive tissues of the body and the crura of the clitoris are embedded deeply near the pubic symphysis and are not removed when excision of the protruding parts take place. Even women with infibulation often have parts of the sensitive tissue of the clitoris and labia left intact. Some studies suggest that, apart from the external genitals, other erogenous zones in the body may become more sensitized in women with genital mutilation, particularly when the overall sexual experience is pleasurable with a caring partner. Also, the psychological and cortical components of the sexual experience in women with genital mutilation are influenced by various factors that are not always predictable. Better designed studies are needed before more light can be shed on the effects of female genital mutilation on women's sexuality.

Effect on men's sexuality

For men who have to live with the genital mutilation of their wives and sexual partners, the experience can also be unpleasant. A woman from Burkina Faso has described how she feels about sex (27):

"For me, sexual intercourse is painful and I find it difficult to find pleasure from sex. It means that my husband has to take great care not to hurt me and has to control himself all the way."

Her husband relates his own experience:

"You can't let yourself go. You have to control yourself to the end. Such moments, contrary to what you might think, are not relaxing."

But the concept of pleasure varies widely between peoples of different backgrounds and cultures, and from individual to individual. In societies where infibulation is the norm, it might be assumed that most men are conditioned to be aroused by a tighter vaginal entrance, by a passive woman or by one who is experiencing pain. In Somalia and Sudan forceful intercourse to penetrate a tight infibulation is hailed as a sign of masculinity and virility (30). Apart from the pain and distress this may cause the woman, the negative experience affects some men, causing them to become impotent. In one reported case, a penile ulcer resulted from repeated forceful attempts at penetration (21). In Egypt, men have claimed that their excessive alcohol or hashish consumption is because they do not find sex satisfying with their mutilated wives (101).

The increased openness in discussing female genital mutilation also reveals the impact of the practice on marital relations. Husbands often seek extramarital sex with women who are not "circumcised" and describe these women as "complete" and "hot" (26). Female genital mutilation may be the underlying cause of strained familial relations which manifest themselves as anger, aggression and ultimately divorce.

Shandall interviewed 300 polygamous men among whose wives only one was "circumcised" (type III) while the others were "uncircumcised" or had undergone type I (15). Some 266 of the men (88.7%) preferred the latter to the former and 60 (20%) had married their second wives only because "they could not keep up with the ordeal of perforating the progressively toughening scars of their wives every time they had babies". Only 36 men (12%) maintained that coitus with an infibulated wife was enjoyable.

4.
Research

Past research

A review of the literature shows that the amount of scientific information on female genital mutilation is relatively small compared to the scale of the problem and the complexity of the factors that contribute to its continuation. Clinical studies on the physical complications constitute the majority of research to date *(15, 16, 18, 21, 23, 29, 81, 84, 88, 102, 103)*.

Studies on the psychological and sexual effects of the practice are patchy and most are designed to yield only limited information *(20, 91, 97, 99)*.

Epidemiological studies on the prevalence of female genital mutilation by type among different populations are available but they vary widely in representation and validity. Demographic and Health Surveys with questions on female genital mutilation have been completed in Central African Republic, Côte d'Ivoire, Egypt, Eritrea, Mali, Sudan, United Republic of Tanzania and Yemen. Other surveys with representative samples but limited geographical coverage are available for Cameroon *(42)*, Chad (unpublished data), Ethiopia *(48)*, Gambia *(50)*, Ghana *(51)*, Kenya *(53)*, Liberia *(54)*, Niger *(56)*, Nigeria *(58)* and Sierra Leone *(20)*.

Some epidemiological surveys have included questions on attitudes and behaviour *(53, 104, 105)*. However, given the limitations of surveys and the impersonal nature of the interviews, the information generated is limited to quantitative reporting of the proportion of those who support or disapprove of the practice, why they hold these beliefs and their future intentions towards their daughters. Other, qualitative studies on female genital mutilation are anthropological documentations of the phenomenon and attempt to construct a social meaning and symbolism that justify its continuation *(96, 106–108)*. There has been little in-depth research on the beliefs, fears and behavioural causes that influence adherence to the practice, the decision-making process within the family, and when and how information against the practice becomes meaningful. The most neglected area is that of applied or operational research on how to design interventions that would convince individuals and communities to stop the practice. Methodologies for monitoring and evaluating different interventions are also lacking. A study from Sudan moves in this direction by assessing the effects of past campaigns and identifying which media and messages were most successful *(109)*. The researchers were partially successful in achieving their stated goals.

Given the social and behavioural factors involved in female genital mutilation it is reasonable to suggest that future research should be focused on behavioural and programmatic aspects of combating the practice. Epidemiological studies are needed to establish baseline prevalence rates. The inclusion of questions on the practice in more Demographic and Health Survey questionnaires will ensure that such baseline data are available for most countries in the near future. Clinical research to quantify the contribution of female genital mutilation to the mortality and reproductive morbidity of girls and women could be useful in influencing policy decisions, and would provide the information base needed for developing clinical support for girls and women who suffer from the health complications of female genital mutilation.

Suggested research agenda

There is clearly a lack of data on the extent, types and effects of female genital mutilation throughout the world, and little research has been undertaken on ways of combating the practice and managing its consequences. This section highlights gaps in current knowledge and provides suggestions for appropriate future research in the following main areas: epidemiology, health effects, behavioural determinants, and programme design and evaluation.[1]

Epidemiology

Epidemiological research should address two sets of questions:

- Is there sufficient evidence that female genital mutilation is practised in the particular country or community to justify taking action?

- What is the scale of the problem: what groups in the country practise female genital mutilation; at what age is it performed; who performs the procedure; and what different methods are used?

---

[1] An in-depth discussion of research issues can be found in *Inroads to behavioral change: a research agenda for female genital mutilation and other reproductive and sexual health issues (110)*.

4. RESEARCH

Prevalence rate

Prevalence rates can be reported by type of procedure, ethnic group, religious following, income, education, age at which female genital mutilation is undertaken etc. Researchers who study female genital mutilation should familiarize themselves with the WHO four-type classification on page 6. Local terminologies and practices should be investigated and matched to this classification. Local variations as to who, how, when and why communities practise female genital mutilation are considerable. Research designed to inform people/organizations carrying out interventions, will therefore need to take into consideration the local factors that influence continuation and those that are the most likely to bring about change in each community. For example, in some countries, ethnic and religious affiliations are currently the most significant causes of continuation, while emerging variables such as parents' level of education, income level, mother's employment, nuclear family structure and female-headed households may influence future decision-making in the family.

Measuring trends over time

Studying the prevalence of female genital mutilation among different age groups through multiple cross-sectional surveys or longitudinal multigenerational studies is the most definitive means of measuring change. However, both of these types of studies, especially the latter, are expensive and require major investments in human and material resources. Since behavioural change in relation to such a deeply rooted practice is expected to be slow, measurable change will be detected only over long periods.

Establishing population at risk at local level

Given the wide variations in the practice of female genital mutilation, exact knowledge of the age at which it is carried out at any particular time and place and of how social trends may shift the practice to a younger or older age is important in order to identify who has escaped the practice and who is still at risk. Such detailed information is useful for the design of interventions to promote behavioural change.

Age-specific prevalence rates

This indicator could measure the incidence of female genital mutilation among an identified population at risk and could be used as a faster measure of trend than multigenerational studies. For example, if the age at which female genital mutilation is performed in a particular community is known to be 4–8 years, the prevalence of genital mutilation among girls in that age group who attend school can be documented. A community-based intervention can be implemented, prevalence in the same age group measured every 2–3 years in the same schools and changes in prevalence rates noted.

The advantage of using age-specific indicators is that the population to be studied may be found in a defined location such as a primary school. Its major drawback is that, unless the age at which genital mutilation is performed and the proportion of girls who attend school remain constant, the measure is not reliable. Another consideration is that the behaviour of families who send their girls to school may be different from that of families who do not, so that the prevalence rate in school may not match that of the general population. In addition, varying school enrolment rates must be taken into consideration.

Despite the limitations, age-specific prevalence rates from the same setting may still prove useful as measures of change over a relatively short period of time.

Health effects

In this category five questions should be addressed. The first relates to the short-term health effects of female genital mutilation, the remaining four to the long-term consequences, namely:

(1) What is the contribution of genital mutilation to the mortality and morbidity of girls?

(2) Do complications of genital mutilation increase the risk of maternal mortality?

(3) What is the contribution of the practice to reproductive morbidity?

(4) What are the effects of genital mutilation on women's psychological and sexual health?

(5) How does genital mutilation affect women's fertility and use of family planning?

To date, the majority of studies on the health consequences of female genital mutilation have been carried out among clients of gynaecology clinics. What is missing is measurement of the contribution of the practice and its complications to the overall morbidity and mortality of girls and women. Although such studies are no longer necessary to justify action against female genital mutilation, they may influence the decisions

4. RESEARCH

of policy-makers towards starting programmes and passing professional regulations or legislation to combat the practice.

Measuring the burden of disease due to female genital mutilation is important and can be used in calculating the cost of this unnecessary practice to the beleaguered economies of Africa and in convincing governments to support abolition programmes.

Mortality in girls

Although some studies and reports document the occurrence of death among girls who have recently undergone genital mutilation (*111*), and there is considerable anecdotal evidence to suggest that it is by no means rare, there has been no systematic investigation of the scale of the problem. Death may be caused by neurogenic shock, immediate severe bleeding or overwhelming infection, and can therefore be easily linked to the procedure. However, later deaths due to slower bleeding, heart failure from severe anaemia or secondary infection may not be attributed to the operation. Several methodologies can be used to measure mortality from genital mutilation in girls, including an adaptation of the "sisterhood method" used for maternal mortality and secondary analysis of survey data collected using questions on the age at which the procedure is undertaken and child mortality. Reliable data on mortality would be most useful to all concerned in designing policies and programmes to combat female genital mutilation.

Morbidity in girls and effect on education

Various degrees of bleeding amounting to haemorrhage are known to be common to all types of female genital mutilation. By the time a girl undergoes the procedure at age 4–16, she may already be anaemic from inadequate nutrition and/or from menstrual blood loss. The acute bleeding following the operation may initiate or exacerbate an already existing anaemia (*102*). Anaemia is known to be a major debilitating condition for girls. Its effects are particularly relevant in the pre-pubertal and early reproductive years, as anaemic children have reduced learning abilities. As a result, genital mutilation may contribute to reduced educational achievement of girls.

Genital mutilation may also affect a girl's education more directly. The ritual may be performed during school days, healing may take a long time or the girl may develop infection or other complications which cause her to miss school. In parts of Kenya, girls are removed from school to undergo the procedure and are then married immediately and not allowed to return to school (53). In such communities, stopping female genital mutilation may reduce the numbers of early marriages. School absenteeism or drop-out due to female genital mutilation needs to be documented through research. Studying the effect of the practice on girls' health and educational achievements is important to programmes for children.

Maternal mortality

Although some correlation between female genital mutilation and maternal mortality probably exists, no studies have provided conclusive evidence to substantiate this. In fact, few studies adequately document the effect of genital mutilation on pregnancy outcomes. In Somalia, it has been observed that some women deliberately starve themselves to reduce the size of the fetus in an attempt to avoid the complications of infibulation (22). However, research on women with malnutrition has shown that the condition has little effect on the incidence of prolonged or obstructed labour. One study reports the possibility of higher incidence of fetal distress among infibulated women. However, the mechanism by which this may occur if the woman has been adequately defibulated is not scientifically obvious nor was any explanation suggested by the study (88). There have been anecdotal reports of stillbirths.

Retention of the products of miscarriage in the vaginal canal has been reported with types II and III female genital mutilation. Obstructed second stage of labour due to tough scars around the vaginal exit is often mentioned but no documented evidence has been found. In fact, since the elasticity of the birth canal itself is not affected by any type of female genital mutilation there should be no reason for obstructed labour. In infibulated women, the most likely outcome would be severe perineal tearing around the narrowed outlet beyond the vaginal introitus if defibulation is not performed. The scar is unlikely to be too tough to be torn by uterine contraction.

Female genital mutilation may contribute to maternal mortality and morbidity through increased risk of bleeding or infection. However, incidents of intrapartum or postpartum haemorrhage or septicaemia solely attributable to it have not been reported. Female genital mutilation and its complications are more likely to add incrementally to other causes of maternal mortality and morbidity than to be the sole causative factor. More detailed information is needed before definitive statements on this subject can be made. Whatever the possible mechanisms, the contribution of genital mutilation to the alarmingly high rates of maternal mortality in Africa needs to be scientifically documented.

4. RESEARCH

Reproductive morbidity

The list of immediate and long-term complications of female genital mutilation, both common and rare, is a directory of reproductive morbidity. Case reports are abundant in the literature and further studies can only add to this information by quantifying its contribution to common conditions, such as reproductive tract infections and infertility.

Psychological effects

The psychological effects are the least explored area of clinical research on female genital mutilation. It is therefore important to investigate the relationship between female genital mutilation, gender inequality and women's subordination. It is also important to look at the role the experience plays in shaping the personal identity and self-image of young women in terms of their right to control their bodies, as their sexuality may influence their reproductive decisions later in life. Understanding the psychosocial dynamics of female genital mutilation may therefore enhance understanding of other reproductive health decisions women make, including health-seeking behaviour and decisions related to childbearing. Other important psychological questions are:

- What are the mechanisms of internalization of social roles which make women accept and defend female genital mutilation?
- Why is it difficult and painful for women to realize the damage done to them through female genital mutilation?
- What counselling and/or support systems do women need to reject the practice and protect their daughters from it?

Finding ways to heal women psychologically will not only benefit them individually, but may be essential to stop them from perpetuating the practice. Unless women recognize and accept the damage done to them and find the means to cope with their own pain they will not attempt to stop female genital mutilation.

It would also be useful to determine whether there is a difference in the social, educational and personal achievement of girls who have undergone genital mutilation compared with those who have not. This question could be answered through case-control studies, with careful attention to possible confounding factors, such as wealth, family status, and rural or urban dwelling.

Sexual effects

More attempts have been made to study sexual effects of female genital mutilation than any other psychological complication. Unfortunately, many reports are unclear in their methodology and conclusions. More studies are needed to explore the effect on the sexual experience of women and men and how that in turn affects the stability of long-term unions. It is equally important to research ways of counselling women with genital mutilation and their partners on how to improve their sexual relationship.

Behavioural determinants

This category of research should look into at least the following questions:

- Why do members of a particular local community practise female genital mutilation?
- What information do they have and what information do they need to help them understand the health risks and human rights violations related to the practice?
- What are the stages of the decision-making process inside the family and how can they be influenced to decide against the practice?
- How can women who have suffered from the practice be helped to accept what has been done to them and empowered to protect their daughters?

Reasons for the practice

Most anthropological and ethnographic studies look into the social meaning of female genital mutilation but do not attempt hypotheses on how to bring about change. These studies contribute insight into the belief systems and knowledge on which the practice is based. They also reveal that the rationalizations used to support the practice vary dramatically between communities. In Egypt, for example, female genital mutilation is performed primarily to preserve premarital chastity (*112*), while among some tribes in Kenya it is a signal that the girl is ready to be sexually active, irrespective of whether she is married or not (*113*). In Sierra Leone, girls may have sexual relationships before they undergo the procedure (*20*). Research to understand the rationale for female genital mutilation in a society is a prerequisite to designing effective messages for change.

Attitudes towards the practice

In terms of attempts to measure attitudes, most of the information in the literature comes from survey questionnaires. The questions asked have not usually gone beyond a simple enquiry about the intention to have daughters "circumcised" and the reasons behind the decision (*21, 53, 103*). While these types of questions can provide useful baseline data for future assessments of interventions, they do not provide information on how interventions should be designed.

Most studies report a much higher number of persons who want to continue than of those who want to stop. This is to be expected, since female genital mutilation is still practised by the majority in those communities where it occurs. Programmatically, however, the more interesting group of respondents are not those who approve of the practice but those who disapprove of it. In the Kenya survey, for example, nearly one-third of the respondents stated that they were against the practice (*53*). The research challenge is to look into the characteristics of this minority and draw lessons from why they changed their attitudes. As allies for change, this group could also be tapped for insider information about determinants of behaviour in the community and about the power and decision-making hierarchies in the family.

Knowledge of the practice and sources of information

Some studies look at current perceptions in the community regarding the benefits and harmful effects of female genital mutilation and whether it is a religious or customary requirement (*109*). No study has looked into how these perceptions developed and where different members of the community go for their information.

More studies are needed to identify local sources of information and to determine which are considered the more trustworthy. The assumption that information usually comes from community leaders such as religious authorities, teachers and doctors may be true in some, but not all, situations. For example, some women may not change their attitude towards female genital mutilation unless they receive the signal of approval from influential women within their support network, regardless of the health or religious evidence presented to them by other authority figures, for it is the women's leaders and their networks who will ensure the good reputation and marriageability of their daughters.

Investigating other social risks involved in behavioural change is important for the design of appropriate interventions. Behavioural change does not occur as a simple and direct response to receiving rational or scientific information. For instance, many doctors continue to smoke despite their knowledge of the harmful effects of the habit. Parents who fear that their daughters will be perceived as promiscuous if they do not undergo genital mutilation will need a stronger motivation to stop the practice than just scientific information. In a society where a woman's chastity is more valuable than her life, health risks become irrelevant. For this reason, it is important to separate chastity as a moral attribute from physical cutting of the genitals. This is a prime strategy of the Egyptian task force on female genital mutilation. Public testimonies by non-circumcised women who are highly respected as role models may be more effective in these communities than health or religious messages (*112*).

Identifying causes of behavioural change

No studies have been undertaken to investigate the reasons why certain individuals, families or communities have stopped practising female genital mutilation. There is a need to study the profile of these social pioneers so they are identified, targeted and recruited as agents of change in their communities. Researchers are currently looking into the experience of a village in the socially conservative region of upper Egypt, where the population stopped practising female genital mutilation because of an intervention implemented by an NGO affiliated to the church. Case studies of families can provide useful information for the design of appropriate interventions and the development of new, more effective messages.

Where a measurable decline in the practice has occurred, it is important to study the role of direct and indirect causes of that decline. Examples of direct causes are specific education and training efforts, media campaigns or personal counselling by health care providers. Indirect causes may include increased levels of female education, improvement in women's economic autonomy, and the effects of urbanization or modernization in shifting the decision-making process to the nuclear family. An attempt should be made to assess the role each factor plays in the ultimate decision to stop the practice.

Programme design and evaluation

Some of the questions to be answered in this regard are:

- Who are the key groups in the family or the community who are likely to change their attitude more readily and how powerful are they in the decision-making hierarchy?

- Who are the best messengers to persuade individuals and communities against the practice? What training do they need and where should they be located?

- How should messages and interventions against female genital mutilation be designed and how can their effectiveness best be evaluated?

4. RESEARCH

- How can changes in the prevalence of the practice best be monitored over time?

Designing effective messages to motivate change

In the past, messages developed for interventions against female genital mutilation were based on the knowledge and untested instincts of members of the community. While these are prerequisites for any such intervention, it is also important to analyse systematically the content and effect of different messages.

Change can be motivated by challenging the perceived benefits of female genital mutilation to those who hold power, such as fathers, uncles, elderly women and other family members. The perceived benefit for girls' morality and health also has to be challenged. Developing messages on the benefits of not practising female genital mutilation to all parties concerned may be a good counter-tactic. These and many other strategies need to be tried and tested.

Operational research

No research has been undertaken on the operational aspects of implementing interventions against female genital mutilation. The desirability, feasibility and means of integrating messages against the practice into school curricula, professional training and individual counselling within the health services is uncharted territory. Educational materials should be developed according to identified needs and their impact should be assessed. Examples of materials developed for these purposes are available, but there has to be more systematic testing of their design and impact.

Economic research

For policy decisions as well as programme priorities, some research on the economic aspects of female genital mutilation is needed. Firstly, it is important to determine whether attempts to persuade practitioners, who benefit both socially and economically, to seek alternative employment have been successful. Some evidence suggests that this approach in relation to a service that is highly in demand may benefit the supplier but may not improve the overall situation since the same suppliers may continue despite alternative training or, even if they stop, other suppliers will step in to fill the demand. In some countries, such as Egypt, the profile of practitioners has changed — current mothers mainly experienced genital mutilation at the hands of traditional practitioners while in the case of their daughters the procedure was undertaken primarily by doctors. Patterns of modernization of the practice have also been reported among affluent families in Nigeria, Somalia and Sudan. While legislation may not affect traditional practitioners who operate outside the formal system, physicians and trained health personnel may be more responsive to legislative measures through fear of losing their license or reputation.

A second area of research is to calculate the economic costs of treating complications and of the burden of disease and disability attributable to female genital mutilation. This could be important in persuading governments to support programmes and legislation to combat the practice.

Evaluation and monitoring

If the abolition of female genital mutilation is to become a reality, each investment in research and each intervention should have a built-in means of measuring its contribution to the ultimate goal of stopping the practice. Evaluation of the efficacy of a particular project and monitoring of the effectiveness of the overall programme against the practice are different exercises which need different approaches and techniques.

Project evaluation is a shorter-term exercise that looks at how a particular project is moving towards its stated goals. For example, a mass education campaign with messages directed at men could be evaluated quantitatively by finding out the number of men who were reached and how many times they heard the message. It can be evaluated qualitatively by finding out how much of the information in the message they retained and whether it had any effect on their attitudes and intended behaviour. Such an assessment may be made at the end of the intervention or at intervals during it.

A project designed to convince the public and policy-makers of the need to pass legislation against female genital mutilation should be evaluated on the basis of its ability to show an effect on public opinion, the views of government officials and the direction of the debate. These are intermediate indicators, while the ultimate measure for this effort is the passing of legislation.

Programme monitoring refers to the effectiveness of all the efforts concerned in reducing the incidence of the practice. As discussed above, the monitoring of change could be partially achieved by measuring the decline in age-specific prevalence rates. Other short-term community monitoring techniques, such as a register of girls who have not undergone genital mutilation, could be developed with the assistance of health workers and community leaders. This type of monitoring was used successfully in one project in Nigeria (58). Monitoring of programmes would also include the documentation of progress of policies, changes in legislation and professional regulations designed to combat the practice, and the amount of financial and human resources invested in abolition efforts. The ultimate monitoring indicator is the decline of female genital mutilation prevalence rates over time. Such monitoring is possible with the integration of questions on female genital mutilation into repeated national surveys, such as the Demographic and Health Survey, which is undertaken approximately every 10 years.

5.
International, regional and national agreements and actions

Female genital mutilation has recognized implications for the human rights of women and children. It is also considered to be a form of violence against the girl, which affects her life as an adult woman. A summary of the international and regional legal instruments which relate to female genital mutilation is available from WHO.[1] These instruments are elaborated further in this section.

International

A series of human rights instruments dating from 1948, which are legally binding on States Parties, contain language concerning the rights to health, non-discrimination on the basis of sex or gender, and physical and mental integrity. Female genital mutilation violates each of these precepts. More recently, language in international conference declarations has directly addressed harmful traditional practices in general and, in some cases, female genital mutilation specifically.

The Universal Declaration of Human Rights, adopted by the United Nations General Assembly in 1948, established a number of basic human rights principles, among them, the inherent freedom and equality of all human beings (*114*, Article 1). Starting from these principles, it sets out a number of basic human rights to which each person is entitled. Article 3 guarantees the right to life, liberty and security of person. This principle has come to be articulated as providing the basis for the right to physical and mental integrity. The Declaration prohibits torture and "cruel, inhuman or degrading treatment or punishment" (Article 5).

The International Covenant on Economic, Social and Cultural Rights and the International Covenant on Civil and Political Rights, comple-

---

[1] *Female genital mutilation.* Geneva, World Health Organization, 1996 (unpublished document WHO/FRH/WHD/96.26; available on request from Family and Reproductive Health, World Health Organization, 1211 Geneva 27, Switzerland).

5. INTERNATIONAL, REGIONAL AND NATIONAL AGREEMENTS AND ACTIONS

mentary human rights treaties adopted by the United Nations General Assembly in 1966 and legally binding on States Parties, have provisions applicable to the practice of female genital mutilation (*115, 116*). The first is the right to self-determination, set out in Article 1.1 of the International Covenant on Economic, Social and Cultural Rights. This guarantees to all persons, *inter alia*, the right to "freely determine their ... social and cultural development". Article 12 of the International Covenant on Economic, Social and Cultural Rights expands the right to health set out in Article 25.1 of the Universal Declaration of Human Rights, declaring that all persons have a right "to the enjoyment of the highest attainable standard of physical and mental health", specifying that States Parties should create conditions amenable to ensuring the provision of prevention as well as treatment of adverse health conditions. The International Covenant on Civil and Political Rights supplements the above, adding that, "Every human being has the inherent right to life", which "should be protected by law" (Article 6). With regard to health and the individual person, it proscribes "torture or ... cruel, inhuman or degrading treatment or punishment" (Article 7). It also expressly prohibits the non-consensual subjection of persons to medical or scientific experimentation (Article 7).

The 1979 Convention on the Elimination of All Forms of Discrimination against Women, legally binding on States Parties, strongly promotes the rights of women and specifically addresses discriminatory traditional customs and practices (*117*). It calls on States Parties to take immediate steps towards eliminating such discrimination by refraining from future discriminatory acts or practices, as well as "to modify or abolish existing laws, regulations, customs and practices which constitute discrimination against women" (Article 2f). Article 5 obligates States Parties to "modify the social and cultural patterns of conduct of men and women, with a view to achieving the elimination of prejudices and other practices which are based on the idea of the inferiority or superiority of either of the sexes or on stereotyped roles for men and women". States Parties are obligated in Article 10 to ensure that women have "access to specific educational information to help to ensure the health and well-being of families". Finally, in Article 12, States Parties are obligated to "take all appropriate measures to eliminate discrimination against women in the field of health care...". The provisions of the Convention, although they do not expressly refer to female genital mutilation, establish a strong international legal basis for the institution of measures to eliminate the practice.

The 1985 Nairobi Forward-Looking Strategies for the Advancement of Women suggest a number of ways in which the international community could promote the rights of women (*118*). Several provisions are applicable to female genital mutilation, although there is no specific reference to the practice. Paragraph 148 calls on governments to establish plans for the promotion of women's health and development to "identify and reduce risks to women's health and to promote the positive health of women at all stages of life". There is a more direct statement against harmful practices in paragraph 150 which states that "health education should be geared towards changing those attitudes and values and actions that are discriminatory and detrimental to women's and girls' health". The same paragraph goes on to state that "steps should be taken to change the attitudes and health knowledge and composition of health personnel so that there can be an appropriate understanding of women's health needs".

The 1993 United Nations Declaration on Elimination of Violence Against Women (*119*) expressly states in its Article 2: "Violence against women shall be understood to encompass, but not be limited to, the following: (a) Physical, sexual and psychological violence occurring in the family, including ... dowry-related violence ... female genital mutilation and other traditional practices harmful to women..." (*119*).

The 1989 Convention on the Rights of the Child, ratified by all states where female genital mutilation is practised, specifically sets out human rights principles applicable to children (*120*). Among other things, the Convention on the Rights of the Child establishes the child's right to develop physically, mentally and socially to his or her fullest potential, to freely express his or her opinion, and to participate in decisions concerning his or her future. Article 19, which protects children from "all forms of physical or mental violence, injury or abuse, neglect or negligent treatment, maltreatment or exploitation", is applicable to female genital mutilation. More specifically, however, the Convention on the Rights of the Child refers to harmful traditional practices in Article 24.3 which states that "States Parties shall take all effective and appropriate measures with a view to abolishing traditional practices prejudicial to the health of children".

A World Medical Association statement on Condemnation of Female Genital Mutilation was adopted by the 45th World Medical Assembly in Budapest, Hungary, in 1993 (*121*). The statement condemns both female genital mutilation and the participation of physicians in the practice.

Building on growing human rights precepts, the 1993 Vienna Declaration and Programme of Action strongly supports the rights of women and girls (*122*). It is applicable to female genital mutilation not only in this way, but also in its specific mention of harmful traditional practices and in its condemnation of them. Reflected in this Declaration is the acceptance by the international community that women's rights are human rights

5. INTERNATIONAL, REGIONAL AND NATIONAL AGREEMENTS AND ACTIONS

and that violence against women is a human rights violation, even if the perpetrator is a private individual or family member. Paragraph 9 states that "the human rights of women and of the girl-child are an inalienable, integral and indivisible part of universal human rights". It goes on to state that "the human rights of women should form an integral part of the United Nations human rights activities including the promotion of all human rights instruments relating to women". Further, the same paragraph declares as priority objectives of the international community the "full and equal participation of women in the political, civil, economic, social and cultural life", as well as "the eradication of all forms of discrimination on grounds of sex". Paragraph 9 then calls for the elimination of gender-based violence and sexual exploitation, including acts and practices "resulting from cultural prejudice", since such acts and practices are "incompatible with the dignity and worth of the human person". It suggests that the international community may achieve the above goals through legal means and other national action, and through cooperation among nations in programmes of economic and social development, including education, health and social support. Finally, the paragraph "urges governments, institutions, intergovernmental and nongovernmental organizations to intensify their efforts for the protection and promotion of human rights of women and the girl-child". Paragraph 10, which addresses the issues of sexual violence and gender bias, expressly calls for "the eradication of any conflicts which may arise between the rights of women and the harmful effects of certain traditional or customary practices, cultural prejudices and religious extremism".

The 1994 Declaration and Programme of Action of the International Conference on Population and Development (ICPD), which strongly advocates gender equity and equality and women's empowerment as well as directly addressing reproductive health and rights issues, make five specific mentions of female genital mutilation and calls for its prohibition (9). The document represents a shift at the international level away from thinking about female genital mutilation primarily as a health issue and towards considering it as an issue of women's health and rights. It also specifically calls for the abolition of female genital mutilation in paragraph 4.22: "Governments are urged to prohibit female genital mutilation wherever it exists and to give vigorous support to efforts among nongovernmental and community organizations and religious institutions to eliminate such practices". Paragraph 5.5 characterizes female genital mutilation as coercive and discriminatory, calling for the adoption and enforcement of measures to eliminate it. Paragraph 7.35 characterizes it as both a "violation of basic rights" and "a major lifelong risk to women's health". This paragraph includes female genital mutilation in a class of harmful practices which were "meant to control women's sexuality" and which have "led to great suffering". Reflecting the status of female genital mutilation as a violation of the right to health, paragraph 7.40 specifically delineates ways in which governments and communities can eliminate the practice. This paragraph emphasizes the urgency of such action and suggests that "steps to eliminate the practice should include strong community outreach programmes involving village and religious leaders, education and counselling about its impact on girls' and women's health, and appropriate treatment and rehabilitation for girls who have suffered mutilation". It adds that such services "should include counselling for women and men to discourage the practice". Finally, paragraph 7.6 states that "active discouragement of harmful practices such as female genital mutilation should also be an integral component of primary health care including reproductive health care programmes".

The 1995 Report of the World Summit for Social Development held in Copenhagen makes specific provisions for the rights of women (Commitment 5) and of the girl child (Commitment 6) (*123*). It also specifically refers to female genital mutilation, reinforcing the ICPD language condemning the practice. In keeping with this, Commitment 6(y) calls for increased international support and cooperation "for education and health programmes based on respect for human dignity and focused on the protection of women and children, especially against exploitation, trafficking and harmful practices, such as child prostitution, female genital mutilation and child marriages".

The Declaration and Platform for Action of the Fourth World Conference on Women, held in Beijing in September 1995, builds on all of this prior action. In addition to strong statements supporting women's and girls' rights, it reinforces the ICPD language calling for an end to the practice of female genital mutilation (*10*). In paragraph 39, which refers to the rights of girls, the document lists female genital mutilation as one of the various forms of sexual and economic exploitation to which girls are often subjected. Paragraph 93 refers to female genital mutilation in the context of social discrimination. It recognizes that conditions "that subject [girls] to harmful practices, such as female genital mutilation" which "pose grave health risks" are common. It goes on to recognize the need for girls to have access to health services, including counselling, as well as access to sexual and reproductive health information. Additionally, this paragraph recognizes that "a young woman's right to privacy, confidentiality, respect and informed consent is often not considered" with respect to health services, and the need for young men to be educated "to respect women's self-determination and to share responsibility with women in matters of sexuality and reproduction".

5. INTERNATIONAL, REGIONAL AND NATIONAL AGREEMENTS AND ACTIONS

Female genital mutilation also receives specific mention in the Platform's section on the strengthening of preventive programmes that promote women's health. The document calls for the United Nations and other relevant international organizations, governments, NGOs, the mass media and the private sector to respect women's health programmes. In paragraph 107(a), which calls for prioritization of various educational programmes for women, the Platform calls for the placement of "special focus on programmes for both men and women that emphasize the elimination of harmful attitudes and practices, including female genital mutilation...".

In the section on equality and non-discrimination, the Platform issues a particularly strong call to governments to ensure, via national constitutions or appropriate legislation, women's equality as well as the elimination of discrimination on the basis of sex (paragraph 232, (a) et seq.). According to section (d) of this paragraph, governments should remove legal provisions not in accord with these principles. Paragraph 232(g) calls for urgent government action to "combat and eliminate violence against women, which is a human rights violation, resulting from harmful traditional or customary practices, cultural prejudices and extremism". Along these same lines, paragraph 232(h) calls for the prohibition of "female genital mutilation wherever it exists", as well as for the "support of efforts among non-governmental and community organizations and religious institutions to eliminate such practices". More generally, various provisions of paragraph 232 call for the implementation of legal and educational measures to ensure the rights of women. Finally, in the section on the girl child, paragraph 259 lists female genital mutilation as an example of gender discrimination, and paragraph 277 calls for the development of "policies and programmes, giving priority to formal and informal education programmes that support girls" as well as placing emphasis on programmes to educate "women and men, especially parents, on the importance of girls' physical and mental health and well-being, including the elimination of discrimination against girls in food allocation, early marriage, violence against girls, female genital mutilation, child prostitution...".

Regional

The African Charter on the Rights and Welfare of the Child, adopted by the Organization of African Unity (OAU) in 1990, protects many of the rights ensured by the Convention on the Rights of the Child (*124*). Article III of the Charter ensures the right to "equality between the sexes". Also applicable to female genital mutilation are Article XIV.1, which ensures that children are provided with the "best attainable state of physical, mental and spiritual health" and Article XVI.1, which gives children the right "to be free from torture and inhuman treatment or child abuse". More directly applicable to female genital mutilation is a provision in Article XXI, which applies to social and cultural practices, requiring governments to "take all appropriate measures to eliminate harmful social and cultural practices affecting the welfare, dignity, normal growth and development of the child...". Harmful practices are specified in the next two clauses, which read: (a) "those customs and practices prejudicial to the child on the grounds of sex or other status"; and (b) "those customs and practices discriminatory to the child on the grounds of sex or other status".

National

According to the opinion of some legal scholars (*125*), female genital mutilation is illegal under any criminal code that punishes bodily injury. However, the lack of will to apply such interpretation to the criminal code and make it applicable to female genital mutilation drives many to call for specific national laws to prohibit the practice. The first country to introduce specific legislation in that regard was Sudan in 1946, under British colonial rule. The law mentions only infibulation, leaving milder forms not punishable by law. The 1993 revision of the Sudanese penal code does not mention any form of female genital mutilation, leaving the legal status of the practice more ambiguous. In 1959, the Minister of Health in Egypt prohibited health professionals from performing female genital mutilation. Given that it is illegal for unqualified health personnel to undertake surgical procedures, the regulation meant that no practitioner was legally allowed to do so. In 1994, another Minister of Health reversed this decree and allowed female genital mutilation to be performed in designated hospitals at a fixed price, arguing that allowing it to be practised under medical supervision would reduce complications. However, as a result the practice became more openly performed and several cases of documented death were reported by the media. In response to a national and international campaign, the 1994 decree was reversed and the current Minister of Health has declared that it is forbidden for health workers to perform female genital mutilation. In 1994, Ghana became the first independent African state to pass a law against female genital mutilation. Burkina Faso and Ghana are among the few African countries with an explicit law prohibiting the practice.

Among countries with African immigrant populations, legislation against female genital mutilation was passed first in Sweden in 1983,

5. INTERNATIONAL, REGIONAL AND NATIONAL AGREEMENTS AND ACTIONS

followed by the United Kingdom in 1985, Australia in 1994 and Norway in 1995. In the United States of America, Congress passed a bill in 1995 requiring the Department of Health and Human Services to support collection of population statistics on African immigrants and to provide educational programmes to inform communities of the harmful effects of female genital mutilation. Further, a federal law prohibiting female genital mutilation has been passed. Eight states have passed specific laws against the practice: California, Delaware, Louisiana, Minnesota, North Dakota, Rhode Island, Tennessee and Wisconsin. There is no specific law against female genital mutilation in Denmark, France or Netherlands, but a case brought to the courts in France in the late 1980s to protect a child against the practice has set a precedent that would make the practice illegal under the criminal code, and the governments of the other two countries have made statements that the practice is illegal under current criminal law. There is no explicit law against female genital mutilation in Italy and Israel.

Ethical considerations

The events in Egypt described above reflect the widespread controversy that exists between proponents of female genital mutilation who believe that a mild form performed by medically trained personnel is a safer option and those who condemn all forms of the practice, no matter how minimal. This debate is common in countries and communities where female genital mutilation is widely practised and among some anthropologists and women's rights advocates in western countries. It is therefore important to establish the scientific facts and ethical grounds on which all types of female genital mutilation must be condemned by the health community. WHO has already condemned all forms of the practice, called for its abolition and unequivocally stated that no form of female genital mutilation should be practised by any health professional in any setting, including hospitals and other health establishments (*11*).

As indicated on page 24, the female genital organs play a vital role in the sexual response of women, and cutting or removal of even a few millimetres of highly sensitive tissue results in substantial damage. The psychological impact of the experience, with its pain and trauma, and the social message that accompanies the ritual have also been discussed. Two of the most important principles of professional health ethics are to do no harm and to preserve healthy functioning body organs at all costs unless they carry life-threatening disease. Female genital mutilation entails the cutting of healthy functioning body organs to comply with a traditional ritual which has no justification on health grounds. It is usually performed on legal minors with no power or faculties to consent. Consent by parents or guardians is not acceptable when the act performed is damaging rather than beneficial to the child. The argument that female genital mutilation performed under hygienic and medically controlled conditions is a lesser evil compared to the greater risk of severe complications is also not acceptable, since the cause of the risk is human behaviour, which can be changed, and not an uncontrollable pathology such as malignancy. Since all medical research and clinical efforts aim at making uncontrollable causes of damage to the human body more controllable, it would be unethical for a health professional to damage a healthy body in order to prevent more destructive human behaviour. It is therefore difficult to find a medico-legal justification for the performance of female genital mutilation on children by health professionals.

6.
WHO policies and activities

WHO started its efforts to promote the elimination of harmful traditional practices in the 1970s. These efforts included gathering information on female genital mutilation, especially regarding its epidemiology and health consequences. These efforts, which are still continuing, include advocacy at international, regional and national levels for the elimination of female genital mutilation. On the basis of research findings, WHO works to promote technically sound policies and approaches to the prevention of female genital mutilation and the management of its health consequences, and to provide support to national networks or organizations and groups involved in developing relevant policies, strategies and programmes. Since the early 1980s, WHO has issued several statements and adopted resolutions on female genital mutilation. These activities and policies are considered below in more detail.

The Seminar on Traditional Practices held in Khartoum, Sudan, in February 1979, which was sponsored by the WHO Regional Office for the Eastern Mediterranean, was the first international forum on female genital mutilation. It took the unprecedented step of formulating recommendations on the elimination of female genital mutilation by governments, including the setting up of national commissions for the coordination of activities aimed at doing this.

In August 1982, WHO made a formal statement of its position to the United Nations Commission on Human Rights, endorsing the recommendations of the Khartoum seminar. WHO's main points were:

— that governments should adopt clear national policies to abolish the practice of female genital mutilation, and to inform and educate the public about its harmfulness;

— that programmes designed to combat the practice should recognize its association with extremely adverse social and economic conditions, and should respond sensitively to women's needs and problems;

— that the involvement of women's organizations at the local level should be encouraged, since awareness and commitment to change must begin with them.

In the same statement, WHO expressed its unequivocal opposition to any medicalization of the operation, advising that under no circumstances should it be performed by health professionals or in health establishments. Together with UNICEF, WHO also stated its readiness to support national efforts against female genital mutilation and continued collaboration in research and dissemination of information.

In the ensuing years, WHO's role included providing technical and financial support for national surveys, for the training of health workers and for grassroots initiatives. For example, WHO supported the NGO Working Group on Female Circumcision which was established in 1977 under the auspices of the Commission on Human Rights to coordinate the actions of NGOs in this area. In 1983, WHO and the NGO Working Group on Female Circumcision convened an informal meeting on the subject with African delegates to the Thirty-sixth World Health Assembly.

In 1984, WHO headquarters and its Regional Offices for Africa and for the Eastern Mediterranean joined UNICEF and UNFPA in providing technical and administrative support and financial assistance to a seminar in Dakar organized by the NGO Working Group on Female Circumcision and sponsored by the Government of Senegal. The Dakar seminar gave further impetus to the establishment of national committees in all countries where female genital mutilation is practised. It set up the Inter African Committee on Traditional Practices Affecting the Health of Women and Children (IAC) to act as a bridge between the groups working among the people and those providing support for their activities.

The efforts of IAC and the NGO Working Group on Traditional Practices Affecting the Health of Women and Children (formerly the NGO Working Group on Female Circumcision) have led to the formation of 24 national committees in Africa that carry out activities for the elimination of this practice with the support of the United Nations and other international funding agencies. WHO continued its support to IAC by cosponsoring the IAC regional seminars on traditional practices affecting the health of women and children in Africa, held in Ethiopia in 1987 and in 1990. The outcome of the 1990 IAC seminar was a proposal for a change in terminology from "female circumcision" to "female genital mutilation". WHO also provided funding to IAC to undertake a comparative study of female genital mutilation and contraceptive use among women in Djibouti and Sierra Leone.

The subject of female genital mutilation, along with other harmful practices, was also discussed during a Regional Workshop on Women, Health and Development, jointly sponsored by WHO, UNICEF and UNFPA in November 1984 in Damascus, Syrian Arab Republic.

In September 1988, the Thirty-fifth session of the WHO Regional Committee for the Eastern Mediterranean passed a resolution on maternal and infant mortality (socioeconomic implications) which stated that women's health must be safeguarded by ensuring the elimination of harmful traditional practices, including female genital mutilation. The WHO Regional Office for the Eastern Mediterranean has also supported the establishment of a regional network of national focal points on women's health through which it supports various activities aimed at the prevention of harmful traditional practices including female genital mutilation.

At its Thirty-ninth session in 1989, the WHO Regional Committee for Africa adopted Resolution AFR/RC39/R9 on traditional practices affecting women and children, recommending that Member States: "(1) prohibit the medicalization of female circumcision and discourage health personnel from performing the operation; (2) include in training programmes for health and traditional birth attendants relevant information on the dangers of female circumcision; and (3) encourage research projects to identify the most effective means of controlling these practices."

WHO participated in a Regional Seminar on Traditional Practices Affecting the Health of Women and Children, organized by the United Nations Centre for Human Rights in Ouagadougou in 1992. The seminar recommended that the terminology "female genital mutilation" be used in the future. In the same year WHO issued a joint statement on female genital mutilation with the International Federation of Gynecology and Obstetrics drawing attention to its harmful effects on health and suggesting approaches for action to abolish the practice (90).

In 1993, the Forty-sixth World Health Assembly adopted Resolution WHA46.18 on maternal and child health and family planning for health which stated that harmful traditional practices such as female genital mutilation "further restrict the attainment of the goals of health, development and human rights for all members of society". Notable here are the changes in language. The stronger and arguably more accurate term "female genital mutilation" is substituted for the term "female circumcision" and there is a recognizable shift from addressing the practice only in terms of a health issue towards acknowledging it as both a health and a human rights issue. The resolution urged Member States to continue the monitoring and evaluation of their efforts to eliminate the practice and requested the Director-General to "collaborate with other organizations and bodies of the United Nations system, governmental and nongovernmental organizations in contributing to the preparation of a plan of action for eliminating harmful traditional practices affecting the health of women, children and adolescents".

The Forty-seventh World Health Assembly in 1994 adopted Resolution WHA47.10 which recognized that traditional practices such as female genital mutilation and early sexual relations and reproduction "cause serious problems in pregnancy and childbirth and have a profound effect on the health and development of children, including child care and feeding". The resolution went on to urge Member States "to assess the extent to which harmful traditional practices affecting the health of women and children constitute a social and public health problem in any local community or sub-group" and "to establish national policies and programmes that will effectively, and with legal instruments, abolish female genital mutilation". It also requested the Director-General to "mobilize additional extrabudgetary resources in order to sustain the action at national, regional and global levels".

In 1995, WHO convened a Technical Working Group on Female Genital Mutilation, which met in Geneva, Switzerland from 17 to 19 July, to draw attention to female genital mutilation and its health consequences, to begin the process of developing standards and norms in relation to the practice and to make recommendations for future action. On the basis of its recommendations, the WHO definition and classification of female genital mutilation reproduced on page 6 was drawn up.

The WHO Regional Office for Africa and UNFPA co-funded the IAC training seminar aimed at strengthening the operational capacity of its national committees, which was held in Burkina Faso in July 1995.

The WHO Regional Office for Africa launched a regional plan of action for accelerating the elimination of female genital mutilation in the countries of the Region in March 1997. WHO also published a joint statement on female genital mutilation together with UNICEF and UNFPA in April 1997 (23).

7.
Conclusion

The centuries-old practice of female genital mutilation used to be shrouded in silence. However, in the past five years that shroud has been removed and female genital mutilation has become one of the most talked about subjects among women's groups, especially in Africa. It is a topic of national and international media attention and most international assistance agencies have developed policies or programmes to combat it. It was an important issue at the World Conference on Human Rights in 1993, a clearly stated violation of reproductive and health rights at the International Conference on Population and Development in 1994 and one of the major issues exposed at the United Nations Fourth World Conference on Women in 1995. Many have reached the conclusion that, recognizing the imbalance of power between men and women that underlies the practice, the most effective strategies for dealing with female genital mutilation include helping women to empower themselves within their own culture and community. Essentially this means that the struggle to stop the practice as a health risk and a violation of women's rights must be led by women from the communities where it occurs. Since Africa is the region where this practice predominates it is natural that African women have been at the forefront of exposing it locally and internationally.

This does not mean, however, that others have no role to play. The support of men and of people from other cultures who are sympathetic to the views of African women opposed to the practice is vital. A number of groups have the potential to provide assistance in this regard.

The international development aid community

International organizations working in Africa and other communities where female genital mutilation is practised have a major role to play. Such organizations can respond to requests for resources (both technical and financial) from local NGOs and government programmes that are opposed to the practice. The limitations of this review do not permit a full report on the policy and funding trends in programmes to combat female genital mutilation over the past 10 years but the overall picture suggests a rapidly rising political interest in the issue with a much slower, and often non-existent, rise in budget for grants or activities. If this trend continues, the current interest in the topic may eventually fade and the practice may once again be shrouded in silence.

International women's groups

Women's groups can help by monitoring progress towards eliminating female genital mutilation and by helping to make sure that resources continue to be available when needed. Women's groups can support the promotion and protection of the health and development of women and girls by listening to what women affected by this practice have to say and by following their lead.

National governments

Some national governments have made a clear and public commitment to stop female genital mutilation through laws, professional regulations and programmes and by signing international declarations that condemn the practice. The launching of the WHO African Region's "Plan of action for accelerating female genital mutilation elimination in Africa" in March 1997 has contributed to a growing interest in the subject among governments. Some have begun developing national policies and plans of action for eliminating female genital mutilation, including setting targets for elimination and developing national-level and district-level indicators for monitoring and evaluating programmes. There is more emphasis on integrating efforts to prevent female genital mutilation into existing health and education programmes and on building partnerships with nongovernmental groups and communities in order to bring about change. Although passing laws to criminalize female genital mutilation may not be appropriate in view of the current stage of development of the movement against the practice in certain countries, it is still important to consider doing so in due course.

National groups

National NGOs, universities and other institutions, and professional associations can help to draw attention to the need to promote and protect reproductive health and to eliminate female genital mutilation. Governments are more likely to take action against the practice when greater numbers of citizens oppose it.

7. CONCLUSION

It is essential to document, review and evaluate approaches and programmes. If activities to combat female genital mutilation are to be successful, the needs and concerns of national groups cannot be ignored.

Finally, it is now possible to believe that the beginning of the end of female genital mutilation is here. Women in Africa and elsewhere, perhaps for the first time ever, have a serious chance of abolishing this humiliating practice while at the same time addressing other problems of discrimination and inequality that they face. With the right approaches locally and sensitive international support, female genital mutilation can and will be defeated.

References

1. Katz J. *The silent world of doctor and patient.* New York, NY, Free Press, 1984.
2. Anderson P. *Children's consent to surgery.* Buckingham, Open University Press, 1993.
3. Declaration of Geneva, 1948. In: *Handbook of declarations.* Ferney-Voltaire, World Medical Association, 1996.
4. Declaration of Helsinki, 1986. In: *Handbook of declarations.* Ferney-Voltaire, World Medical Association, 1996.
5. Declaration of Tokyo, 1975. In: *Handbook of declarations.* Ferney-Voltaire, World Medical Association, 1996.
6. Wolkoff AS. Surgery of the clitoris. In: Lowry, TP et al. *The clitoris.* St Louis, MO, Warren H. Green Inc., 1976:104–110.
7. Hosken F. The epidemiology of female genital mutilation. *Tropical doctor*, 1978, 8:150–156.
8. Taylor JR, Lockwood AP, Taylor AJ. The prepuce: specialized mucosa of the penis and its loss to circumcision. *British journal of urology*, 1996, 77:291–295.
9. *Programme of action.* Cairo, International Conference on Population and Development, 1994.
10. *Declaration and platform for action.* Beijing, Fourth World Conference on Women, 1995.
11. *Female genital mutilation. Report of a WHO Technical Working Group, Geneva, 17–19 July 1995.* Geneva, World Health Organization, 1996 (unpublished document WHO/FRH/WHD/96.10; available on request from Family and Reproductive Health, World Health Organization, 1211 Geneva 27, Switzerland).
12. Daniell WF. On the circumcision of females in West Africa. *Medical gazette of London, England*, 1847:374–378 (Cited in: Huelsman BR. An anthropological view of clitoral and other female genital mutilations. In: Lowry TP et al. *The clitoris.* St Louis, MO, Warren H. Green Inc., 1976:111–161).
13. Roles RC. Tribal surgery in East Africa during the 19th century: Part two — Therapeutic surgery. *East Africa medical journal*, 1967, 44:17–30 (Cited in: Huelsman BR. An anthropological view of clitoral and other female genital mutilations. In: Lowry TP et al. *The clitoris.* St Louis, MO, Warren H. Green Inc., 1976:111–161).

REFERENCES

14. Worsley A. Infibulation and female circumcision: a study of a little-known custom. *Journal of obstetrics and gynaecology of the British Empire*, 1938, 45:686–691.
15. Shandall AA. Circumcision and infibulation of females: a general consideration of the problem and a clinical study of the complications in Sudanese women. *Sudan medical journal*, 1967, 5:178–212.
16. Verzin JA. Sequelae of female circumcision. *Tropical doctor*, 1975, 5:163–169.
17. Daw E. Female circumcision and infibulation complicating delivery. *The practitioner*, 1970, 204:559–563.
18. Aziz FA. Gynecologic and obstetric complications of female circumcision. *International journal of gynaecology and obstetrics*, 1980, 17:560–563.
19. El Dareer A. *Women, why do you weep?* London, Zed Press, 1982.
20. Koso-Thomas O. *The circumcision of women: a strategy for eradication.* London, Zed Press, 1987.
21. Dirie MA, Lindmark G. The risk of medical complications after female circumcision. *East African medical journal*, 1992, 69:479–482.
22. Johnson KE, Rodgers S. When cultural practices are health risks: the dilemma of female circumcision. *Holistic nursing practice*, 1994, 8:70–78.
23. *Female genital mutilation: a joint WHO/UNICEF/UNFPA statement.* Geneva, World Health Organization, 1997.
24. Iregbulem LM. Post-circumcision vulval adhesions in Nigerians. *British journal of plastic surgery*, 1980, 33:83–86.
25. Diejomaoh FME, Faal MKB. Adhesions of labia minora complicating circumcisions in the neonatal period in a Nigerian community. *Tropical geographical medicine*, 1981, 33:135–138.
26. Kere LA, Tapsoba I. Charity will not liberate women. In: *Private decisions, public debate.* London, Panos Press, 1994.
27. Toubia N. *Female genital mutilation: a call for global action*, 2nd ed. New York, NY, RAINB?, 1995.
28. Dirie MA. Female circumcision in Somalia: medical and social implications. In: *Proceedings of the SOMAC/SAREC (Sweden) Conference, Mogadishu, Somalia, 1985.*
29. Mustafa AZ. Female circumcision and infibulation in the Sudan. *Journal of obstetrics and gynaecology of the British Commonwealth*, 1966, 73:302–306.
30. Van der Kwaak A. Female circumcision and gender identity: a questionable alliance. *Social science and medicine*, 1992, 35:777–787.
31. Modawi S. The impact of social and economic changes in female circumcision. In: *Proceedings of the Third Congress of Obstetrics and Gynaecology, Khartoum.* Khartoum, Sudan Medical Association, 1973:242–254 (Sudan Medical Association Congress Series, No. 1).
32. *Sudan fertility survey.* Khartoum, Department of Statistics, Ministry of Economic and National Planning, 1979.
33. Sudan Ministry of Economic and National Planning & Institute for Resource Development/Macro International. *Sudan demographic and health survey, 1989/1990.* Calverton, MD, Macro International, 1991.

34. Hosken F. *The Hosken report*, 1st ed. Lexington, MA, Women's International Network News, 1979.
35. Toubia, N. *Female genital mutilation: a call for global action*. New York, NY, RAINB♀, 1993.
36. Toubia N. Two million girls a year mutilated. In: *The progress of nations*. New York, NY, UNICEF, 1996.
37. *The world's women*. New York, NY, United Nations, 1995.
38. *World population prospects: the 1994 revision*. New York, NY, United Nations, 1994.
39. *Enquête et témoignages sur la pratique de l'Excision en République du Bénin (Survey and evidence of the practice of excision in the Republic of Benin)*. Porto-Novo, National Committee on Harmful Traditional Practices, 1993 (unpublished report).
40. Nitiema PA. *Les mutilations génitales féminines dans la ville de Ouagadougou: épidémiologie — évolution. (Female genital mutilations in the town of Ouagadougou: epidemiology — evolution)*. Ouagadougou, University of Ouagadougou Faculty of Health Sciences, 1993 (unpublished thesis).
41. Lamizana M, Comité National de Lutte contre la Pratique de l'Excision. Update on female genital mutilation in Burkina Faso. In: *Report of the Second Annual Inter-agency Working Group Meeting on female genital mutilation*. New York, NY, RAINB♀, 1995.
42. Njock Nje Y et al. *Research on female genital mutilation in Cameroon*. Yaoundé, National Committee on Harmful Traditional Practices, 1994 (unpublished report).
43. Central African Republic, Ministry of Economics, Planning and International Cooperation/Macro International. *Enquête démographique et de santé, République Centrafricaine 1994-95. (Demographic and health survey, Central African Republic 1994–95)*. Calverton, MD, Macro International, 1995.
44. Côte d'Ivoire Ministry of Economics, Finance and Planning/Macro International. *Enquête démographique et de santé, Côte d'Ivoire, 1994 (Demographic and health survey, Côte d'Ivoire, 1994)*. Calverton, MD, Macro International, 1995.
45. Warzazi A. *Report of the Working Group on Traditional Practices Affecting the Health of Women and Children*. New York, NY, United Nations Economic and Social Council, Commission on Human Rights, 1991.
46. Saadawi N. *The hidden face of Eve*. London, Zed Press, 1977.
47. Assaad M. Female circumcision in Egypt: social implications, current research and prospects for change. *Studies in family planning*, 1980, 11:3–16.
48. Gebere Selassie A, Desta M, Negesh Z. *Harmful traditional practices affecting the health of women and children in Ethiopia*. Addis Ababa, Ministry of Health/UNICEF, 1984.
49. Meskal FH, Dijene A, Yuduhfa A. *Perceptions and attitudes regarding harmful traditional practices in Ethiopia*. Addis Ababa, National Committee on Harmful Traditional Practices/Ministry of Health, 1990.

REFERENCES

50. Singhateh SK. *Female circumcision, the Gambian experience: a study on the social, economic and health implications.* Banjul, The Gambia Women's Bureau, 1985.
51. Kadri J. *The practice of female circumcision in the upper east region of Ghana: a survey report.* Accra, Ghanaian Association for Women's Welfare, 1986.
52. Twumasi PA. *Female circumcision in selected areas in southern Ghana.* Accra, Ghanaian Association for Women's Welfare, 1987.
53. *Report on harmful traditional practices that affect the health of the women and their children in Kenya.* Nairobi, Maendeleo ya Wanawake Organization, 1991.
54. Marshall R et al. Traditional practices affecting the health of women and children in Liberia. In: *Seminar on traditional practices.* Dakar, Inter-African Committee on Harmful Traditional Practices Affecting the Health of Women and Children, 1984.
55. Republic of Mali, Ministry of Health, Solidarity and Aged Persons/Macro International. *Enquête démographique et de santé, Mali, 1995–96: Rapport préliminaire. (Demographic and health survey, Mali, 1995–96, preliminary report).* Calverton, MD, Macro International, 1996.
56. Salamatou T et al. *Enquête primaire sur les pratiques traditionnelles ayant effets néfastes sur la santé de la mère et de l'enfant au Niger. (Primary survey of traditional practices with harmful effects on mothers and children in Niger).* Niamey, Comité Nigerien de lutte contre les pratiques traditionnelles néfastes, 1992.
57. Issa B. *Communication concernant l'excision au Niger (Communication on excision in Niger).* In: *Réunion préparatoire de la conférence régionale sur l'excision. (Preparatory meeting for the regional conference on excision).* Ouagadougou, National Committee on Harmful Traditional Practices, 1993 (unpublished document).
58. Adebajo C. Update on female genital mutilation in Nigeria. In: *Report of the Global Action Against Female Genital Mutilation first inter-agency working group meeting on female genital mutilation.* New York, NY, RAINB♀, 1994.
59. Mottin-Sylla M-H. *L'excision au Sénégal: éléments d'information pour l'action. (Excision in Senegal: elements of information for action).* Dakar, Environnement et Développement du Tiers-Monde (ENDA), 1990.
60. Abdalla R. *Sisters in affliction: circumcision and infibulation of women in Africa.* London, Zed Press, 1982.
61. *Female circumcision: strategies to bring about change. Proceedings of the International Seminar on Female Circumcision, Mogadishu, Somalia, 13–16 June 1988.* Rome, Somali Women's Democratic Organization/Italian Association for Women in Development, 1989.
62. *Female genital mutilation in Uganda.* Geneva, Inter-African Committee on Traditional Practices Affecting the Health of Women and Children, 1993 (IAC video).
63. *Report of the IAC Regional Conference, Tanzania, 1990.* Geneva, Inter-African Committee on Harmful Traditional Practices Affecting the Health of Women and Children, 1991 (unpublished document).

64. Hedley R, Dorkenoo E. *Child protection and female genital mutilation: advice for health, education and social work professionals.* London, FORWARD Ltd, 1992.
65. Harel D. Medical work among the Falashas of Ethiopia. *Israel journal of medical science,* 1967, 3:483–490.
66. Grisaru N, Lezer S, Belmaker RH. Ritual female genital surgery among Ethiopian Jews. *Archives of sexual behavior,* 1997, 26 (2):211–215.
67. Asali A et al. Ritual female genital surgery among Bedouin in Israel. *Archives of sexual behavior,* 1995, 24:573–577.
68. Ghadially R. Update on female genital mutilation in India. *Women's Global Network for Reproductive Rights newsletter,* January-March 1992.
69. Srinivasan S. Behind the veil, the mutilation. *The Independent (Times of India), Sunday,* 14 April, 1991 (magazine section, "Vantage").
70. Pratiknya AW. Female circumcision in Indonesia: a synthesis profile for cultural, religious and health values. In: *Female circumcision: strategies to bring about change. Proceedings of the International Seminar on Female Circumcision, Mogadishu, Somalia, 13–16 June 1988.* Rome, Somali Women's Democratic Organization/Italian Association for Women in Development, 1989.
71. Gilbert SG. *Pictorial human embryology.* Seattle, WA, University of Washington Press, 1989.
72. Stilwell DL. Anatomy of the human clitoris. In: Lowry et al. *The clitoris.* St Louis, MO, Warren H. Green Inc., 1976:9–21.
73. Lowry TP. Some issues in the histology of the clitoris. In: Lowry et al. *The clitoris.* St Louis, MO, Warren H. Green Inc., 1976:91–97.
74. Sillah MM. Bundu trap. *Natural history* (the monthly magazine of the American Museum of Natural History), 1996, 105:42–51.
75. United Press International. Press notice, 25 August 1996.
76. Asuen MI. Maternal septicaemia and death after circumcision. *Tropical doctor,* 1977, 7:177–178.
77. Warsame A. Social and cultural implications of infibulation in Somalia. In: *Female circumcision: strategies to bring about change. Proceedings of the International Seminar on Female Circumcision, Mogadishu, Somalia, 13–16 June 1988.* Rome, Somali Women's Democratic Organization/Italian Association for Women in Development, 1989.
78. El Dareer A. Epidemiology of female circumcision in the Sudan. *Tropical doctor,* 1983, 13:41–45.
79. Silberstein AJ. Circoncision féminine en Côte d'Ivoire. (Female circumcision in Côte d'Ivoire). *Annales de la Société Belge de Médicine Tropicale,* 1977, 57:129–135.
80. Fleischer NKF. A study of traditional practices and early childhood anaemia in Northern Nigeria. *Transactions of the Royal Society of Tropical Medicine and Hygiene,* 1975, 69:198–200.
81. Sami I. Female circumcision with special reference to the Sudan. *Annals of tropical paediatrics,* 1986, 6:99–115.

REFERENCES

82. Hathout HM. Some aspects of female circumcision with case report of a rare complication. *Journal of obstetrics and gynaecology of the British Empire*, 1963, 70:505–507.
83. Post MTH. *Female genital mutilation and the risk of HIV*. Soutien pour l'Analyse et la Recherche en Afrique (SARA) Issue Paper, May 1995.
84. Rushwan H. Etiologic factors in pelvic inflammatory disease in Sudanese women. *American journal of obstetrics and gynecology*, 1980:877–879.
85. Brown Y, Calder B, Rae D. Female circumcision. *Canadian nurse*, 1989, 85:19–22.
86. Agugua NEN, Egwuatu VE. Female circumcision: management of urinary complications. *Journal of tropical pediatrics*, 1982, 28:248–252.
87. Onuigbo WIB, Twomey D. Primary vaginal stone associated with circumcision. *Obstetrics and gynecology*, 1974, 44:769–770.
88. DeSilva S. Obstetric sequelae of female circumcision. *European journal of obstetrics, gynaecology and reproductive biology*, 1989, 32:233–240.
89. McCaffrey M. *Female genital mutilation: consequences for reproductive and sexual health*. London, British Association for Sexual and Marital Therapy, 1995:189–200.
90. World Health Organization, International Federation of Gynecology and Obstetrics. Female circumcision, female genital mutilation. *International journal of gynecology and obstetrics*, 1992, 37:149.
91. Baasher TA. Psychological aspects of female circumcision. In: *Fifth Congress of Obstetrical and Gynaecological Society of Sudan*. Alexandria, World Health Organization Regional Office for the Eastern Mediterranean, 1977.
92. Bijleved C. *The effect of education on Sudanese women's attitudes towards female circumcision*. Leiden, University of Leiden, 1985.
93. Grassivaro Gallo P, Moro Moscolo E. Female circumcision in the graphic reproduction of a group of Somali girls: cultural aspects and psychological experiences. *Psychopathologie Africaine*, 1985, 10:165–190.
94. Sanderson LP. *Against the mutilation of women: the struggle to end unnecessary suffering*. London, Ithaca Press, 1981.
95. Lightfoot-Klein H. The sexual experience and marital adjustment of genitally circumcised and infibulated females in the Sudan. *The journal of sex research*, 1989, 26:375–392.
96. Boddy J. *Wombs and alien spirits. Women, men, and the Zar cult in northern Sudan*. Madison, WI, University of Wisconsin Press, 1989.
97. Megafu U. Female ritual circumcision of Africa: an investigation of the presumed benefits among Ibos of Nigeria. *East African medical journal*, 1983, 60:793–800.
98. Lightfoot-Klein H. Pharaonic circumcision of females in the Sudan. *Medicine and law*, 1983, 2:353–360.
99. Karim M, Ammar R. Female circumcision and sexual desire. *Ain Shams medical journal*, 1966, 17:2–39.
100. Badawi M. Epidemiology of female sexual castration in Cairo, Egypt. *The truth seeker*, July/August 1989, 31–34.
101. Karim, M. *Circumcisions and mutilations: male and female*. Cairo, The National Population Council, 1994.

102. Egwuatu VE, Agugua NEN. Complications of female circumcision in Nigerian Igbos. *British journal of obstetrics and gynaecology*, 1981, 88:1090–1093.
103. Olamijulo SK et al. Female child circumcision in Ilesha, Nigeria. *Clinical pediatrics*, August 1983, 580–581.
104. El Dareer A. Attitudes of Sudanese people to the practice of female circumcision. *International journal of epidemiology*, 1983, 12:138–144.
105. Dirie MA, Lindmark G. Female circumcision in Somalia and women's motives. *Acta obstetrica et gynecologica scandinavica*, 1991, 50:581–585.
106. Gruenbaum E. The Islamic movement, development and health education: recent changes in the health of rural women in Central Sudan. *Social science and medicine*, 1991, 33:637–645.
107. Gordon D. Female circumcision and genital operations in Egypt and Sudan: a dilemma for medical anthropology. *Medical anthropology quarterly*, 1991, 5:3–14.
108. Skramstad H. *The fluid meanings of female circumcision in a multiethnic context in Gambia: distribution of knowledge and linkages to sexuality*. Fantoft, Norway, Development Research and Action Programme (DERAP), Chr. Michelsen Institute, Department of Social Science and Development, 1990 (Working Paper D).
109. El Nagar SEL, Pitamber S, Nouh I. *Synopsis of the female circumcision research findings*. Khartoum, Babiker Badri Scientific Association for Women Studies, 1994.
110. *Inroads to behavioral change: a research agenda for female genital mutilation and other reproductive and sexual health issues*. New York, NY, RAINB♀ (in press).
111. Dirie MA, Lindmark G. A hospital study of the complications of female circumcision. *Tropical doctor*, 1991, 21:146–148.
112. Assaad M. A harmful practice embedded in culture and tradition. In: *Report from the Seminar on Female Genital Mutilation, Copenhagen, May 1995*. Copenhagen, Ministry of Foreign Affairs/DANIDA, 1996.
113. Ng'ang'a L. Female genital mutilation activities in Africa: focus on Kenya using a case story. In: *Report from the Seminar on Female Genital Mutilation, Copenhagen, May 1995*. Copenhagen, Ministry of Foreign Affairs/DANIDA, 1996.
114. *Universal Declaration of Human Rights*. New York, NY, United Nations, 1948 (United Nations General Assembly resolution 217 A(III)).
115. *International Covenant on Economic, Social and Cultural Rights*. New York, NY, United Nations, 1966 (United Nations General Assembly resolution 2200 A(XXI)).
116. *International Covenant on Civil and Political Rights*. New York, NY, United Nations, 1966 (United Nations General Assembly resolution 2200 A(XXI)).
117. *Convention on the Elimination of All Forms of Discrimination against Women*. New York, NY, United Nations, 1979 (United Nations General Assembly resolution 34/180).

REFERENCES

118. *The Nairobi Forward-Looking Strategies for the Advancement of Women.* Nairobi, World Conference to Review and Appraise the Achievements of the United Nations Decade for Women: Equality, Development and Peace, 1985.
119. *UN Declaration on Elimination of Violence Against Women*, December 1993 (United Nations General Assembly document A/RES/48/104).
120. *Convention on the Rights of the Child.* New York, NY, United Nations, 1959 (United Nations General Assembly resolution 1386 (XIV)).
121. *World Medical Association Statement on Condemnation of Female Genital Mutilation.* Ferney-Voltaire, World Medical Association, 1993.
122. *Vienna Declaration and Programme of Action.* New York, United Nations, 1993.
123. *Report of the World Summit for Social Development.* New York, United Nations, 1996.
124. *African Charter on the Rights and Welfare of the Child.* Addis Ababa, Organization of African Unity, 1990.
125. *Intersections between health and human rights: the case of female genital mutilation.* New York, NY, RAINBØ, 1996.

Recommended further reading

Women's health: WHO position paper. Geneva, World Health Organization, 1995 (unpublished document WHO/FHE/95.8).

Female genital mutilation: information pack. Geneva, World Health Organization, 1996 (unpublished document WHO/FRH/WHD/96.26).

Violence against women: information pack. Geneva, World Health Organization, 1997 (unpublished document WHO/FRH/WHD/97.8).

Gender and health: technical paper. Geneva, World Health Organization, 1997 (unpublished document WHO/FRH/WHD/97.39).

Copies of these unpublished documents are available on request from Family and Reproductive Health, World Health Organization, 1211 Geneva 27, Switzerland.